Who am I in a Traumatised and Traumatising Society?

GREEN BALLOON PUBLISHING

Professor Dr Franz Ruppert, is Professor of Psychology at the University of Applied Sciences in Munich, Germany. He gained his PhD in Work and Organisational Psychology at the Technical University of Munich in 1985.

His publications in English include: *Trauma, Bonding & Family Constellations: Understanding and Healing Injuries of the Soul* (2008), *Splits in the Soul: Integrating Traumatic Experiences* (2011), *Symbiosis & Autonomy: Symbiotic Trauma and Love Beyond Entanglements* (2012), *Trauma, Fear and Love; How the Constellation of the Intention Supports Healthy Autonomy* (2014), *Early Trauma: Pregnancy, Birth and First Years of Life* (2016), *My Body My Trauma My I: Setting up Intentions, Exiting our Trauma Biography* (2018), all published in English by Green Balloon Publishing, Steyning, UK.

Ruppert has spent the last 25 years studying the phenomenon of traumatisation and developing a method of working with unconscious and very early trauma. His theoretical developments come under the title Identity-oriented Psychotrauma Therapy (IoPT).

He teaches his theories and his practical work in Germany and many other countries including Brazil, Austria, Norway, Singapore Switzerland, Britain, Ireland, Italy, Russia, Netherlands, Poland, Portugal, Romania, Turkey and Spain, furthering his insights into the pervasive effects of trauma, while exploring his developing ideas practically using his own method: The Intention Method.

About this book

This book is a personal exploration of Ruppert's Identity-oriented Psychotrauma Theory as it relates to his own life history and his thoughts on our place in society.

The question he poses through this book is: what to do about our society at this seeming crisis point? Professor Ruppert makes his specific focus the dynamics of perpetration and victimization as the cyclic forces that hold us in a continually traumatising and re-traumatising world that it is hard to step away from. His solution to look at ourselves personally and deal with our own unresolved trauma, which allows us to see more clearly each situation in which we are challenged, and to understand what realistically each one of us can do.

His final answer is: we are our society, and if we take ourselves and our own trauma seriously and address the dilemmas within, we will then attract to us the society we want.

Who am I in a Traumatised and Traumatising Society?

How perpetrator-victim-dynamics determine our life, and how we can break free

Franz Ruppert

Translated by Andrea Dalton

Edited by Vivian Broughton

GREEN BALLOON PUBLISHING

First published in the United Kingdom in 2019
by Green Balloon Publishing

German edition first published under the title
Wer bin Ich in einer Traumatisierten Gesellschaft?
by Klett-Cotta

Green Balloon Publishing, Steyning
www.greenballoonbooks.co.uk

ISBN 978-0-9559683-9-6

Book production by The Choir Press, Gloucester
Set in Times

Contents

Preface   xi
Acknowledgements   xv
English Language Editor's Preface   xvii

1. **Humanity and I**   1
    Paradise on earth would be tangibly close   1
    Humanity on the brink of the abyss   4

2. **The human psyche – as inside so outside**   6
    Needlessness, pleasure principle or learning through
    reward?   8
    The pharmacological promise of salvation   10
    Conscious and unconscious psyche   11
    The discovery of bonding and psychotrauma   11
    Human psyche and reality   12
    Memory and remembrance   14
    Shared consciousness   16
    Pseudo realities   17
    Sending and receiving   19
    Healthy psyche   20
    Who am I?   20
    Identifications   21
    Attributions   22
    Demarcations   23
    True identity   24
    To be   25
    Being the subject   26
    To be myself   27
    Healthy, stressed, and traumatised psyche   28
    The boundaries of self awareness   30
    The illusion of psychological health   31
    Hardware and Software   32
    Preservation of the species or the self?   33

Contents

3. Psyche and Society 34
Psychological knowledge is important for all of us 34
Are parents for or against children 38
The absence of maternal affection 39
Education for or against children? 40
Rivalry between men and women 42
Economic competition 45
Political and national rivalry 50
Natural disasters would suffice 53
Constructiveness or destructiveness? 54
To fight or adapt? 56
Existence or consciousness 58

4. Traumatic personal experiences 60
Body-psyche split 61
Trauma Triad 63
Trauma induced splitting of the psyche 64
Surviving instead of living 67
The Psychotrauma Biography 67
The trauma of identity 68
The trauma of love 74
The trauma of sexuality 76
The trauma of becoming a perpetrator 79
Existential trauma and the trauma of loss in the
context of the trauma biography 81
Trauma as the cause of self-destructiveness 82

5. The perpetrator-victim dynamic 85
Psychotrauma-victims 85
The perpetrator of psychotrauma 86
Being the victim 89
Victim-attitude as trauma survival strategies 90
"Those who do not work ... 93
Victim identity 98
From trauma victim to perpetrator 100
Victim attitudes as collective trauma-survival strategies 102
Being a perpetrator 103

Perpetrator attitudes   105
Secrecy and looking away   109
Perpetrator ideologies   110
Perpetrator identity   112
Trauma perpetrators in power   114
The accomplices   116
What do perpetrators of trauma get out of it?   116
To be perpetrator and victim all-in-one   117
The perpetrator-victim split and the body   122
Suicidal tendencies   123
Case study of Anders Bering Breivik: From childhood
trauma-victim to mass murderer   123

6. **Traumatised and traumatising societies**   **130**
    The whole of society fights the symptoms   136
    Effects and repercussions of psychotrauma   139
    Trauma-denying society   140
    How to live in traumatised societies?   142

7. **How attempts to step out fail**   **145**
    Revenge   145
    Rebellion   146
    Revolution   146
    Forgiveness   148
    Reconciliation   149
    Saving other people   150
    Pathologising   151
    Religion   152
    Spirituality   153
    Art   153
    Drug consumption   154
    Rational discourse   155
    Society's failure to recognise the real problems   156

Contents

8. How can we escape?   **158**
The feeling of victimhood ...   158
How to escape from our perpetrator attitudes   161
Psychologically healthy children mean healthy
societies   162

9. IoPT and The intention method   **164**
Angelika:That is where I want to go   166
The practice of intention-work   167
Andreas: I would like to know what it is in me
that I want to kill   168
Perpetrators who trigger their own traumas   169
To remain true to oneself   170
Life beyond the perpetrator-victim dynamic   172
From the healthy 'I' to the healthy 'We'   173
Leadership by compassion   175
What connects us all   177
I am the society   178

References   **179**

Preface

Why am I writing this little book? It started for me in early 2017, as the international situation grew more acute with wars in Iraq, Syria, and Libya, and the resulting, and continuously rising, flow of refugees coming to Germany from Afghanistan, Iraq, Syria, and Africa.

The election of Donald Trump as president of the USA, and the rise of dictatorship in Turkey, the right-wing nationalist movement in France, the Netherlands, and Germany, the threat of nuclear war between North Korea and the United States, just to mention the obvious and, for me, particular threats.

It takes my breath away to witness how, since the end of World War II, shamelessly and cold-heartedly 'World War III' is continuously discussed and promoted as a peacekeeping operation. How the concept of 'enemies' is persistently constructed and held onto. How every escalation of the war between the USA, together with its NATO allies and the former USSR (now Russia) is heralded as a defensive measure. How also now China is becoming a global player in the insanity of competition to produce more and more weapons of mass destruction.

I found I could no longer sleep easily; I noticed how my thoughts increasingly circled around these social and global realities. The level of stress within me kept increasing, and I asked myself what I could do about it.

Therefore, after many years of research and personal work in psychotherapy, I thought that I should make the knowledge that I had acquired on this topic public. So that people might finally wake up and stop persistently traumatising each other so senselessly, and not become further entangled with the insanity of perpetrator-victim dynamics through war and terrorisation, and not force everyone into the final abyss of a nuclear catastrophe.

I was born in 1957 in a small farming village. A broken

portrait of Hitler sat in the attic of my maternal grandmother's house; an ominous pistol lay in my mother's eldest brother's bedside locker; scary war films in black and white on the newly acquired television – I did not understand much in my childhood about the last Great War on German soil. How traumatised my parents were through their parents, the Nazi-dictatorship, and immediate wartime experiences, only became clear to me much later. Moreover, how much my traumatised parents then traumatised me I have only vaguely been able to comprehend and feel in recent years.

I am fortunate enough to be able to work on my own psychotrauma uninterruptedly, and I now no longer doubt the fact that I was not wanted, not loved, and not protected from violence in my childhood.

One restless night in the summer of 2017, during which my body became increasingly tense and I could not sleep, I heard a voice in my ear: "You are allowed to cry!" Suddenly tears streamed from my eyes and from one moment to the next, I completely relaxed. Apparently, this sentence had pacified the small child in me, who had been rejected and beaten whenever he cried or expressed his feelings some 60 years ago. As an infant, I had already learned to suppress my fear of violence and loneliness, my anger, rage, and pain. No longer was I able to scream or cry, but instead I felt ashamed whenever I was not good enough in the eyes of my parents or teachers. My outer appearance had seemed calm, but my inner stress kept increasing.

Attachment researchers call this kind of behaviour 'insecure-avoidant': the child appears calm in order to stay close to his rejecting and punishing parents. Internally he (or she) – I have varied the usage of 'he' or 'she' for general purposes throughout – is under extreme tension, and has to suppress his need for contact and love, always keeping his feelings under control. Recognising this pattern in myself not only pacified me, but also allowed me to feel intensely; after all I had been giving lectures and speeches on this topic for years. Despite an international situation that continues to descend into insanity, I find I can now sleep better than ever before.

I observe something similar in other people: their (childhood) traumas are constantly triggered by present day societal events (terror attacks or dictatorial politicians). They feel panic, become restless, anxious and stressed. However, when they finally take the opportunity to deal with their own childhood traumas they can become calm and regulate their emotions better. Even though this does not change the external world at all, it allows the person to return to their healthy senses and perceive their options and choices more realistically.

None of us can 'save the world', and perhaps we should be particularly cautious of those who try. Every one of us has only a short snapshot of life within an unimaginable dimension of time and space, and we should, therefore, protect this personal precious life from harm. We can even enjoy it as far as the respective international situation and our own life resources allow in the actual moment. We can protect ourselves from the insanity of other people as far as that is possible for us. However, in order to be able to do this we have to learn something important in our work with our own traumatised psyche, so that we do not allow ourselves to be constantly pulled into the vortex of perpetrator-victim dynamics of others that can so easily be established within ourselves.

The fundamental question "Who am I, and what do I want?" includes the consideration "In what kind of community of people do I want to live?" What connects me to my fellow human beings? What separates me from them? Does a 'we' worth spending my vital energy on actually exist? Or is this 'we' merely an illusion of what seems to be a harmoniously regulated, but artificially created, community that is surrounded by and can only exist in discord with other such communities?

Personally, I continue to follow my own path privately and professionally as much as I can. I perform my therapeutic and public work, which I consider accurate and meaningful, and which I enjoy. I find pleasure in witnessing other people finding a similar path, and being helpfully aided in their everyday life. It reassures me that this is a good path. I enjoy my encounters and exchanges with such people. Now I find I can relinquish the company of those who are stuck in perpetrator-victim dynamics without the fear of becoming isolated. I also no longer want to spend time vigorously examining their self-constructed problems.

Ultimately, I have written this little book for myself, in order to organise my own feelings, thoughts and experiences further, and gain clarity about what is most important for me to know about this world and the people assembled on it, to clarify what is socially viable and what is not. It is my intention to avoid the many perpetrator-victim dynamics embedded in traumatised and traumatising societies all around me as much as possible, and not foster any new perpetrator-victim dynamics myself.

That is why I do not want this book to invite anyone into a perpetrator-victim dialogue with me. I am not seeking to lay blame, but to name causes, as I understand them now. I am happy to enter into an exchange with those readers who would like to share their personal experiences in response to my writing. I am pleased when my insights serve to make a contribution and possible transformation towards trauma-free and constructively oriented communities. I can only change myself for the better. If many other people also do that, societies will change, too.

Munich, February 2019

Acknowledgements

Translating a book and preparing it for publication takes many hands and heads to make it possible. So I am grateful to Andrea Dalton for her careful translation of the text; to Vivian Broughton who edited the translation excellently and designed the cover; to John Mitchell for his co-ordination and copy editing; to John Mc Clean for his proofreading; and to Miles Bailey and his team at the Choir Press for their work in bringing the book to publication.

Last but not least I thank all those who allowed me to present their case studies in this book.

Franz Ruppert
Munich 2019

English Language Editor's Preface

As the Editor of this English language version of *Wer bin Ich in einer Traumatisierten Gesellschaft?* I am pleased to be able to be part of the team that presents this book to you. Andrea Dalton of Sussex University handled the translation from German to English, and I thank her for her hard work. The topic is daunting, and the text complex, and her work is greatly appreciated. I also want to thank Simon Lys who helped me with the initial editing of the text.

I hope the readers find the topic interesting and useful, and the book a comfortable read ... that is the aim of an editor: to offer a text that maintains the tone and character of the author, and at the same time provides the English language reader with a text that is accurate to the original and a good read.

Vivian Broughton
London 2019

1
Humanity and I

Paradise on earth would be tangibly close

Humanity as a species ('homo sapiens') has come a long way. In 2018, 7.5 billion people live on this planet – and it is continuously increasing. Such a successful expansion, however, is more of a catastrophe for the diversity of species on earth. A birth rate of 2.0 instead of 2.4 would already lay the foundation for an ecological improvement. Homo sapiens have spawned fantastic cultural and technological achievements, providing themselves with food, clothes, housing, and an infinite variety of products, mobility, and endless information. To be human and to live as a human can be pleasurable and wonderful. Unlimited knowledge is at our disposal. There are extraordinary teachers, educational institutions and learning techniques. There are many people, who are devoted to supporting each other, liking nothing more than to help each other. We can see this every time a natural disaster causes tremendous hardship: immediately there are people on site who are committed to helping.

I see us humans as one part of evolution. Since evolutionary processes always find more or less successful compromise solutions for problems and conflicts, we, too, as Homo sapiens are in many ways also a formula of compromises. We are of average height and average strength. We are of average speed and average intelligence. Even for us humans our natural surroundings are not perfect: we can bear hot and cold conditions only up to a certain point. Even as omnivores, our naturally existing food supplies are limited. Predisposition is the price we have to pay for the advantages of sexual reproduction. Women have to carry the burden of pregnancy, birth and feeding babies. Men's hormonal predisposition involuntarily forces them to rival other men, and they lack the deep emotional bonding to their own child that comes naturally to women due

1

to pregnancy and childbirth. Sexual reproduction causes numerous conflicts of interest between men and women, parents and children, and amongst men and women themselves.

Essentially no one ever has it easy in life because of such challenges for the survival of the self and of the species. The demands on each individual just to live, creating and maintaining new human life, are high, and can drive them to the limits of their abilities. This already provides sufficient meaning and purpose to life, but on closer inspection, we can see that people make each other's lives much more difficult than is necessary for the simple survival of the species and the self. Humans put themselves under enormous pressure, and at times cause immense stress to others, and yet it is not at all apparent how this contributes to their own happiness and joy in life.

In a world that continues to be technologically connected, I can be in touch with friends, colleagues and business partners in Singapore, Brazil, Los Angeles or Moscow in seconds with the help of a mobile phone and the internet. When I want to know something, it only takes a few clicks on the computer and in no time at all I have access to facts and opinions on the topic. In Munich where I live, I have an extensive network of personal relationships, an enormous range of educational institutions, good job opportunities, beautiful cultural events, and culinary delicacies in abundance.

Nevertheless, I find it difficult to enjoy all of this without reservation. For instance, I find it difficult to eat meat when I consider the breeding conditions of chickens, pigs and calves (Safran Foer, 2010). Even though I have not quite become a vegetarian yet, I am close. Also it does not feel good to know how well off I am in comparison to the many millions who do not have a roof over their heads, live from hand to mouth, or merely vegetate and suffer the wretchedness of war in refugee camps.[1] I feel nauseous, and sometimes get angry, when I look at the media and become aware of the daily madness in this world, the destructive goals for which

---

[1] Approximately 65 million people are currently fleeing from imperialism, nationalism, sexism, and capitalism.

people use their time, energy and intelligence, so much money, and so many natural precious resources. The extent of human stupidity, stubbornness, hypocrisy, and power-hunger – which unfortunately is alive in more than just a few people – frightens me.

If only a fraction of the current expenditure of dictatorial leaders on the military, secret services, weapons, and pointless economic wars would be spent on education, health and renewable energy, the whole of the planet would soon be a zone of peace and prosperity for everyone.

Material wealth can easily make us overlook how miserable our inner world is. Professional success, our home space, and our family can blind us to our deep unhappiness, loneliness and feelings of abandonment in this world. Images of the world's poor and oppressed, who are materially considerably worse off than most of us, further distract from the perspective of the internal plight of such middle class citizens. Consequently, for those that have it, material wealth induces feelings of guilt, and provokes the urge to help others. Some dig deep into their pockets whilst others turn helping into a profession; however, most of the time this fails to address properly the underlying causes of external hardship of the poor, or our own internal suffering.

Images of external wealth, on the other hand, create the illusion for the world's poor that rich countries are paradise on earth. Images of such material excesses attract them; that is why many embark on dangerous journeys to desired destinations, even at the risk of losing their lives. Once at their destination they then discover how much mistrust, hostility, and lack of human warmth exist there; that they are only welcome if they somehow manage to make themselves useful, for example as cheap labour.

I, myself, refused to acknowledge my own internal, psychological problems for 50 years. I preferred to keep my focus on other people and social issues. To focus on my own situation was considered to be a narcissistic self-indulgence in the left-wing circles in which I lived as a student. There was no time for it in the fight against the capitalist, imperialistic, and false consciousness for a fairer world of all the others. How traumatised and incapable of maintaining any kind of relationship we ourselves were was a forbidden subject of discussion.

Humanity on the brink of the abyss

War reigns on many battlefields even as we speak. Ruthless competition rages in the economy. Life for many partners and families is also in a state of war. Even on the internet and in social media – where we could actually learn from each other at great speed – often there rage battles of words. Many people send out messages of hate continuously. Axel Hacke (2017) provides an easy to read and absorbing examination on the topic. The most brutal and violent videos are disseminated. A hidden fight with virtual viruses and spyware in order to to hack or destroy others' computers and penetrate their private sphere takes place. In this way, too, human lives are destroyed, and countless people are psychologically terrorised.

There is no hope for those who think that hatred, envy, and oppression are the immutable human destiny determined by the laws of nature, or even God's divine intention. We can only wait until the human species makes itself extinct, or if provoked by their search for military success and short-term profit the forces of nature sweep them off this globe. The climate catastrophe is in full swing, and the means of self-destruction already in place. Approximately 16,300 atomic warheads exist, capable of turning the entire planet into a lifeless desert within minutes, and causing the death of all complex life. Instead of diffusing and scrapping these weapons of madness, they are currently being further 'modernised' by nations with nuclear power – what a cynical term!

Why do people subjugate each other, if good cooperation could be a viable option? Why do people inflict violence on each other if peaceful solutions would so obviously be much better for everyone? Why do people drive each other to insanity, when rational approaches would be much more time and energy efficient? Why will they not stop until they physically and psychologically ruin not just everyone else, but also themselves?

In the recent past humanity has found itself close to global self-destruction several times. For example in the Cuban crisis in the 1960s, and again today in Syria, when the USA and Russia with their supremacy ambitions collide on a fiercely contested battleground. Now even a small country like North Korea joins the madness and threatens the 'enemy' with nuclear annihilation. The following threat alert in Hawaii that spread through mobile phones on Saturday, 13th January 2018, could have easily triggered a nuclear catastrophe in view of the massive tensions between the USA and North Korea: "EMERGENCY ALERTS – BALLISTIC MISSILE THREAT INBOUND TO HAWAII. SEEK IMMEDIATE SHELTER. THIS IS NOT A DRILL."

Even in earlier centuries, people were no less brutal to themselves and others; however, in the last hundred years we have developed the technological potential that allows for total destruction from our blindly inquiring minds. Paradise or hell – in the end this decision may be made by an unstoppable technical algorithm programmed by someone with the best intentions (Harari, 2017).

2
The human psyche – as inside so outside

As human history shows, the reason that determines whether we live a good life, or whether we become a nuisance to each other, lies not so much in our natural environment as within ourselves. For example, people went to war not because of hunger and food shortages, but because of religious and economic reasons, or the personal ideologies of troublemakers and warmongers (Harari, 2015). Even material wealth and the meeting of basic needs for food, drink, clothing, and shelter do not automatically lead to a greater satisfaction with life, or to a peaceful cohabitation.

Whether we humans are cooperative or aggressive depends in the first instance on the state of our psyche. Whatever our psyche looks like, so we fashion our social and natural environment. If chaos reigns within our psyche, we organise chaos in our external world. If we are at peace within our psyche, we can establish clear and orderly conditions in our environment: as inside, so outside.

If that is the case then there is at least a glimmer of hope for our social communities. At least this way we would know what we can/could work on collectively. We would have to:

- learn to understand our human psyche better, and ...
- collectively and individually work on this ...

in order to utilise our psyche for life enhancing rather than destructive intentions, for our own well-being and benefit.

Essentially, our human psyche is a fantastic tool. It has enormous capacity and potential. It can serve us very well as long as we nurture and care for it as something precious, delicate and valuable. It is not predetermined at birth through 'genes',

6

but influenced through our relationships and lifestyle (Bauer, 2002). Therefore, if our psyche is influenced by negative experiences in life, violent relationships, poisoned by unbearable feelings and misled by misunderstandings, our psyche can and must be constantly readjusted.

If we want to lead a better life and not continue to fight each other, we have to gain a better understanding of why the human psyche is so easily entangled in aggressive disputes in our interpersonal relationships. Why does the psyche invest so much energy in escalating perpetrator-victim dynamics instead of searching for constructive solutions? We have to learn how to free ourselves from these endlessly destructive loops. We should not allow or accept becoming slaves of our damaged psyche!

I am certain now, due to extensive work with people in my psychotherapy practice, and from examination of my own psyche, that the crucial reason for human destructiveness is the traumatisation of our psyche. The traumatised psyche leads to endless perpetrator-victim relationship dynamics. If we understand, acknowledge and recognise this fact, a way out of this cycle of destructiveness becomes available, even if it has been in place for a long time and we are habitually used to it. We can learn to be at one with ourselves, and meet other people with goodwill and sympathy even if we have endured much suffering in our life, and inflicted suffering on others.

The prerequisite for this is the willingness to confront our own psyche and our personal history. This requires the company of like-minded people on the same journey. Significant also are the methods that can help us fully understand our psyche, heal it from its injuries, and keep it healthy. These techniques do exist now. With the 'intention method' I have developed a very useful tool with which to explore our psyche, and face the traumas contained within. Generally, the aim is to find a way of becoming constructive when we have lost ourselves in destructive relationships.

Individuals are responsible for their willingness to confront their own psyche. In that area nobody can be forced. Once we have made this fundamental decision we will certainly find people who support us on our journey, and who in turn may benefit from our help.

Needlessness, pleasure principle, or learning through reward?

For some time now religious leaders, philosophers and psychologists have tried to answer the question: what impels us humans to do what we do? What makes us happy and what makes us suffer? Siddhartha Gautama, the founder of Buddhism, saw in our thinking and behavioural processes the main obstacle for a happy life. Therefore, he advised us to free ourselves from all things that induce suffering: the emotional attachment to our needs and ideas that never allow us to be satisfied, and always wanting more. Instead of trying to change feelings that surface now and again and then disappear, he recommended simply leaving them be, not to take them seriously, and dismiss both past and future. For that, he developed numerous meditation techniques, for example paying conscious attention to our breathing.

In the Western world, Sigmund Freud (1856-1939) considered it to be the 'pleasure principle' that we all followed. He said that we constantly strive to experience pleasure and avoid the unpleasurable. With the help of this principle individuals should at least be able to take care of themselves. In the wake of the First World War, and a looming Second World War however, Freud grew increasingly pessimistic. At the end of his life he believed that not just 'Libido' and 'Eros' were at force in the human being (to live and to love), but also 'Thanatos', an unconscious urge that leads us individually and collectively to stupor, death, and doom. "The fateful question of the human species seems to me to be whether, and to what extent, the cultural process developed in it will succeed in mastering the derangements of communal life caused by the human instinct of aggression and self-destruction." (Freud, 1979, page 128). For Freud the ideal way to liberate the individual from 'neuroses', leading to a better existence, was to apply depth psychology in the confrontation with our experiences, especially those from a frustrating childhood. He had no idea what to do regarding society as a whole, "since nobody has the authority to impose this therapy onto the masses." (ibid)

The response of behavioural psychologists to the question "why do we do what we do?" was a little different. They thought that we strive for rewards and avoid punishment. Because of that, we would quickly learn what rewards us ('positive reinforcement'), and refrain from all those things that we see as punishing us ('negative reinforcement'). According to Frederik B. Skinner (1904-1990), one of the founders of this theory, this principle can be of optimal use in getting people to do what the authorities define as 'desirable behaviour'. His political vision of the use of this form of learning theory on the whole of society is given literary expression in his novel "Walden Two" (Skinner, 1972).

Doubtlessly reward and punishment can motivate people to change, at the very least, their expressed attitude. However, this then opens the floodgates for human manipulation: only those who have authority, power and money can define what is 'desirable' and 'undesirable' behaviour, usually according to their own interests, and then condition others until they become accustomed to it and believe that there is no alternative. A report in the "Süddeutsche Zeitung" from 19 May 2017 indicates that the Chinese government has scientists working on the development of a point system for each citizen, which identifies and evaluates them publicly as good or bad. By merging all kinds of electronically stored data, the academics involved in the project consider this to be a real and nationwide possibility in China. By the help of face detection software and Big Data, George Orwell's Vision of "Big brother is watching you!" is now reality – and not only in China.

Without an inner authority that decides to uphold certain behaviour despite punishment, every person could be completely controlled through external influences. However, evidently there is such an inner authority in all humans, and it can be quite resistant to external reward and punishment. This is proven by the examples of young habitual offenders, or drug addicts, or those young girls who voluntarily join the Islamic state in Syria or Iraq and become the architects of their own downfall. In fact neither punishment nor reward will deter some people from crimes, drug use, or shooting innocent people. Luckily, people with clarity of feeling and thought and a healthy self-esteem cannot be so easily impressed and manipulated by reward and punishment either. They know what they want and what they do not want and act of their own accord.

The pharmacological promise of salvation

Spiritual practices and psychotherapy in whatever form demand an engagement with the self, with one's own feelings, thoughts, attitudes, and behaviour patterns. Would it, therefore, not be simpler, less time-consuming and less demanding to obtain the desired changes through psychoactive substances? Indeed this has been a human dream for thousands of years. To swallow, drink, inhale, or inject powerful chemical ingredients and in an instance the world seems, at least temporarily, all right again. Alcohol, Ayahuasca, 'bath salts', cannabis, mushrooms, heroin, cocaine, LSD, nicotine, peyote cacti ... the list of psychoactive drugs is long, and it is added to by whatever substances are concocted every day by the pharmaceutical industry. They enter the market as psychotropic drugs and are sold at high profit as Benzodiazepine, Ritalin, Seroquel etc.

Nevertheless, experience has shown that the effects of such substances are short-lived, and in fact in the end they often cause the opposite of what they are intended for, as the human brain takes countermeasures. This creates the need to increase the dosage leading to drug and medication dependence. The initial 'psychological disorder' turns into 'mental illness'; 'neuroses' and 'psychoses' become chronic, and the psyches of such people fail to develop further (Ruppert, 2002).

Conscious and unconscious psyche

Buddhism and the great and significant schools of psychology and therapy of the 20th century have one fundamental understanding in common: neither the internal experience nor the external behaviour of humans can be controlled through conscious mind and reasoning, but rather our actions are led by unconscious psychological processes that we do not notice at all. The unconscious is that which fundamentally exists beyond conscious sensory perception (images, sounds, smells). It is also what we actively repress and banish from our consciousness. The human consciousness is only a quasi-bonus to those psychological processes that take place beyond our conscious awareness, mental processes, and memories. That is why we have to include the unconscious part of our psyche in our investigation of our behaviour and perceptions in our attempts to change. We have to invite our unconscious to reveal itself and make itself accessible to an enlightened verbalisation. Rational analyses alone are of no further help; indeed they could induce the opposite, vastly strengthening unconscious emotional resistance.

The discovery of bonding and psychotrauma

Since the times of Freud and Skinner, psychologists and psychotherapists have discovered much more about our psyche. In particular, they have identified the emotional bonding process that keeps infants and small children in a symbiotic relationship with their mothers (Bowlby, 1969/2006). Added to the basic understanding of our primal needs, such as food and sexuality, came the realisation that the need for body contact and closeness are also primal instincts and desires. The human species would cease to exist if sexual drives did not continue to prevail. However, the need for emotional closeness and love cannot be excluded or regarded as merely disruptive irrationalities in interpersonal relationships. Physically experienced love is as vital for everyone as his or her daily bread. When love is suppressed in a parent-child or couple relationship we cease to be the higher developed lifeform that humans are; we revert to the level of primitive predators.

As far as I am concerned, after bonding and attachment, psychotraumatology is the second biggest discovery of modern times (Seidler, Freyberger and Maercker, 2011). When medical doctors talk about 'trauma' they refer to injuries of the body through physical or chemical causes (pressure, fire, acid etc). When psychotherapists adopt the term, they are not so much denoting physical injuries, but rather psychological injuries. In the last 50 years psychologists and psychotherapists have gained a much greater understanding of how our life experiences, often traumatising for human perception, feelings, thinking, remembering, and action, affect those concerned. Psychotrauma can pathologically alter our body, and poison human co-existence (Herman, 2003; Levine, 2010; Ruppert & Banzhaf et al, 2018).

The clearer we come to understanding these processes the more obvious it becomes that the ideal of the enlightenment – that everything improves with rational thought and action – is not the key to personal happiness and the wellbeing of societies. Even material reward and professional success cannot compensate for psychological deficits. Ideas such as 'prosperity' or 'employment for all' by themselves do not create harmoniously functioning societies, as capitalist ('liberal', 'market-economy based'), socialist ('social democratic', 'communist'), or nationalist ('republican', 'patriotic') ideologies would have us believe. Even looking at 'environmental issues' through 'green' politics distracts us from our own internal state. Not only flora and fauna are under threat; we are in a crisis ourselves!

Human psyche and reality

The principle function of the human psyche is to make the reality within which a person exists accessible:

- Reality Level 1 is the external world: the concrete ('objective') world consisting of physical and biological factors. So, the earth, the creatures that live on it, and the universe beyond.

- Reality Level 2 is our internal subjective world, as a reflection of the objective world, including the individual's relationship to their surroundings, their environment, to nature and the ties that bind every human to all other living beings.
- Reality Level 3 is the self-constructed world within the psyche that does not exist in level 1 at all.

The human psyche commands several input channels simultaneously, which we call perception. These are the five basic senses; seeing, hearing, smelling, tasting and feeling. These give us our first impression of what is available in our external world. With this, however, we have to remember that our perception is selective based on our individual needs and interests. We never perceive everything that exists; that would not only be an excessive demand on our psyche, but it would also be pointless.

The next psychological processing stage is the feelings we have about what we perceive. Here are the basic emotions: fear, anger, grief, pain, happiness, revulsion, shame, guilt, pride and love. Feelings are the subjective reaction to perceived reality. Human feelings provide an intense contact with the body. They develop through chemical processes in the body that 'messenger' substances regulate. They appear and disappear again more slowly than the processes of perception, which the electrical activities in the brain produce.

The subsequent psychological processing stage gives us the concepts we have of the world, based on our perceptions and feelings. This view of the world could be accurate, or it could miss the real world by a long shot. It is more likely to be wishful fantasies than a recognition of what is actually true.

Only thinking processes can free people from their limited and often anthropocentric worldview. In thinking, we can abstract particularities of our perception, and the subjectivity of our feelings, and draw conclusions beyond them. This can lead to an increasingly accurate recognition of reality as it is. At best this is a generally valid perspective, and thus as correct and true for others as it is for me. Since thinking is based on electrical processing of stimuli, thoughts can quickly appear and disappear, and can be replaced by new ones. Thinking is mostly free from physical metabolic processes, however this may result in the illusion that the mind is not connected to the body.

In addition, the human psyche possesses two significant special functions that are to a great extent missing in other lifeforms: the 'I' and the will. In the course of human development, an increasingly autonomous 'I' can develop in the human psyche, and with that an increasingly clear awareness of our 'I' (Bauer, 2015). Through the 'I' the human being obtains an inner point of reference for perception, feeling, thinking, remembrance, and action. The awareness of this 'I' allows further options for self-reflection, the development of a conscious will, and the focused pursuit of a self-transforming process, for example within the context of psychotherapy.

The human psyche is constantly developing. It selectively serves our needs, can adapt well to external circumstances, and is essentially creative. In other words, time and again it can find good solutions for practical problems. The idea that 'mental illness' cannot be changed because it is genetically determined is scientifically archaic, and no longer corresponds to current knowledge of the nature of the human psyche, the brain, and genetics (Bauer, 2002).

Memory and remembrance

Humans store their experiences, and are able to remember them. This serves their learning ability and the development of their personality. Recollections of experienced realities, like perception, are subjective and selective, and we notice particularly those experiences that are emotionally relevant to us. They make us aware of what scares us, and what makes us happy. The storage of memory content takes place in various areas of the brain, in the (sensory) organs, in the muscles, and in the individual cells. This is why memories are present on several levels of the human organism. The conscious recollection of images, voices, or smells is only a small part of what we can remember.

Much of what we have experienced is unconscious, and stored within us as our body's reaction patterns to certain events. This is why in my experience we even remember prenatal experiences, for example surviving an attempted abortion, and this is why unconscious memories can be awakened. So memory researchers make a differentiation between explicit memories – in other words consciously wanted memories – and implicit memories, which emerge unintentionally (Levine, 2015).

The fact that we cannot remember an event consciously does not mean that we have not experienced it. The event could have occurred before our consciousness was fully developed, or it could have been repressed from our consciousness because it frightened us too much or made us feel ashamed.

Some experiments show that conscious memory recall is not always particularly reliable, and that we can even be persuaded to believe that we have experienced something in which we did not take part (Shaw, 2016). These results are often used to suggest that people are being talked into sexual traumatisation by therapists (Loftus and Ketcham, 1994). Certainly, this cannot be completely excluded, however such experiments often also prove the opposite: no one can be certain that they have not experienced sexual trauma in their childhood, simply because he or she does not have any conscious and clear picture of it. As long as we do not want to remember something consciously, and possess sufficient 'I'-strength, it is always possible that it did happen. In my opinion, this is also due to a lack of memory research. Human memory cannot be studied independently of the person's entire psyche. Memory is part of the psyche and, particularly with experiences that are traumatic, it is of significance whether the person wants to remember the experience or not. The withdrawal of the person's 'I' from the trauma experience is in most of the cases with which I am familiar the preferred trauma-survival strategy. Therefore, if I am not there consciously, and I unconsciously refuse to remember, I can be deluded into thinking that I did not experience a trauma.

At the beginning of my therapeutic practice, I considered the exposure of sexual traumatisation to be the key for psychological healing. In the course of my career, it became increasingly clear that psychological traumatisation is infinitely more complex than this. As I will show later, sexual traumatisation is generally the result of what precedes it: to have been rejected and not loved in childhood. I also had to learn caution when memories of traumatic events and possible connections surfaced in someone triggered by process feedback. Ultimately only the person concerned can sense, feel, and know what was inflicted on them and what their experience was. Therapy can only open up approaches and offer explanations for symptoms. The people themselves have to make their own decisions as to which issues are important to work on, what to expand on, and what should, even must, remain unexplored at the moment. As a rule of thumb, however, I would offer the following hint: physical symptoms are often indicators of traumatic memories.

Many claim that they cannot remember particular periods of their childhood. What to do with this knowledge? Should we be satisfied with it and let the matter rest, or should we be alarmed by it and try to fill the gap? However, people with memory gaps that are trauma related cannot be complete in their identity, and so cannot properly answer the question "Who am I, and what do I want?" Therefore, it requires a conscious decision to bring light into one's own dark past. The memories are there if we want them to show up.

Shared consciousness

On the one hand, the human psyche's understanding and remembering of realities is an individual process. On the other, it is also a link to what our fellow humans recognise as reality. We learn from each other; we process our images of reality collectively. In positive cases, this can lead to mutual support in understanding truths and realities and avoiding being misled. In negative cases it can be that everyone is collectively mistaken, do not want to know the truth, and support each other in that.

That is why I prefer group therapy. For a therapist it is easier to mislead one person who seeks support from him than for a whole group – as long as the group pursues the objective of exposing realities and truths that have been unconsciously hidden. I know now that the human psyche can only be healthy, i.e. function healthily, if it can recognise reality as it was and how the person experienced it, even if that is frightening and painful. That is why I try, together with group participants, to enable every person working on his psyche to recognise his biographical reality, as much as this is possible at any given moment.

Pseudo realities

A further distinctive feature of the human psyche that must not be ignored is that it can invent its own entire world, detached from objective and subjectively processed reality. That is what I call Reality Level 3: the self-constructed world. This only exists in the psyche that is in the mind of the person, in other words what the person considers the world to be is nothing more than his own 'head-birth'.[2]

It is frequently the case that a person cannot differentiate their psychologically self-created reality from the other two levels of reality. Therefore, they insist that their 'head-birth' is the objective reality, thus forcing their 'head-birth' onto themselves and others. In the end, they live completely in their fictitious ideas and delusions, trying to make them true at the expense of actual reality. This subjugation to one's own mental constructs comes at a high price. Potentially, such people subordinate their entire lives to serving the constructs of their own imagination (figure 1).

Unfortunately, this happens quite frequently, for example in the idea of a particular god that everybody is meant to believe in. People are forced to abide by his presumed commands and prohibitions, with brute force if necessary.

Even the idea of a single true and sacred economic system,

---

[2] Taken from the novel by Günter Grass, *Headbirth: the Germans are dying out.*

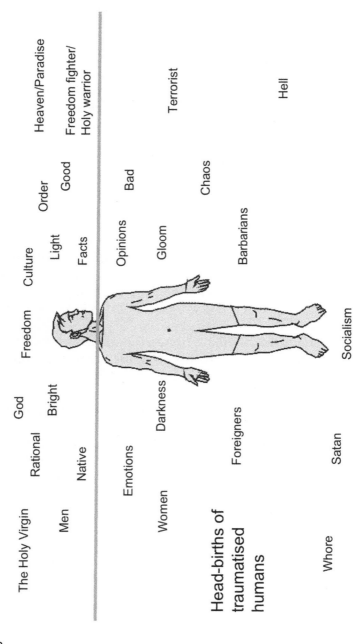

Figure 1: The two-dimensional world of human 'head-births' (reality level 3)

the 'market economy' can be a head-birth; for example, 'capitalism' has been enforced globally over the last 200 years without giving consideration to the actual people and their resulting social interaction. As Alfie Kohn brings it to the point: "Capitalism works to the principle of the glazing trade in which the workers smash windows at night so during the day they can praise their services to the public." (Kohn, 1989, S. 88)

Now purely arbitrary mathematical systems consisting of nothing more than numbers and the way they are offset, like interest rates or stock prices, determine the fate of the whole of humanity (Harari, 2015, p. 374 ff.).

In the private sphere the idea of 'family-honour' can cause great damage in those people who believe, or rather are forced to believe in it by means of verbal brainwashing, and are not allowed to doubt the idea (Said, 2017).

The tendency to believe more in fantasy, illusions, and head-births than to trust one's own perception, feelings, and thoughts is massively encouraged by the suffering of psychotrauma.

Sending and receiving[3]

At its core, the psyche consists of information. As we know from computer technology, one computer can transmit information data packets very quickly to another. That requires a sender, a transmitting channel, and a receiver. The same is true for psychological information. Like data packets, they can be transmitted from one person to the next: Person A sends and Person B receives, if he is online to receive. The electromagnetic waves that our eyes and ears can pick up are the transmission channel. However, there seem to be other and many more transmission channels that so far have been given little attention. In general, they are mostly seen as an obscure form of 'telepathy', and assigned to the field of esotericism.

My experiences with the resonance method over the last 20 years show me that psychological data are not just consciously

---

[3] See chapter 9

transmitted from one person to the next in speaking and writing, but are also unconsciously transmitted without the awareness of sender or receiver. Even people who do not know each other can exchange unconscious information, if they give each other permission to do so, and if their psyche and organism are receptive, as is the case in the resonance process. During a private session of my own, a resonance-giver spoke of green fields, through which he could navigate his way, and he spoke of fences and gates that he could open and close, describing it as a world in which he would keep his herd together, and that it would not be something he could do with his family. I was completely flabbergasted by this, since the resonance-giver could not have known that my father worked as a shepherd when I was a child.

If that can happen with strangers, this exchange of unconscious psychological information, then how much more such psychological information transfer can occur between two people who are close to each other and live together, especially between mothers, fathers, and their children?

Healthy psyche

What does a healthy psyche have to be able to do? It has to be able to ...

- reliably differentiate between the internal and external worlds,
- differentiate between past and present,
- separate 'I' (my experiences) from 'You' (your experiences),
- distinguish between reality and illusion.

Without these prerequisites, psychological disorders will develop: we project our fears into our environment; we live emotionally more in the past than in the here and now: we become entangled with our children, our partners, our friends, our customers. We walk around in illusionary worlds.

Who am I?

The experiences in my psychotherapeutic practise have led me to devote my attention to the development of the 'I', and the question of human identity. For many years I considered that which people describe as their 'I' to be their actual 'I'. Only through the technique of working with intention-statements did I realise the extent to which the 'I' of a person can overlap with the 'I' of another, specifically a perpetrator, especially in situations where the person's own father or mother is the perpetrator. The same holds true for our will. Traumatised people are often not aware that their entire will is adjusted towards the will of the perpetrators who have traumatised them. Instead of living in their own real identity, they live in a symbiotic entanglement with the very people who have traumatised them.

Identifications

The first group of false assumptions in connection with identity are what I have called identifications. Since the real 'I' and the will have to be abandoned early many people initially answer the question "Who am I?" with the following:

- I am a German (an American, a Turk, a Russian ...)
- I am a Christian (a Muslim, a Jew ...)
- I am a doctor (a worker at the XY company, a business employee of YZ)
- I am the child of ...
- I am the husband/wife of ...
- I am a Gemini (Leo, Aries, Pisces ...)

However, these are not statements about their identity but types of identifications. Identification is something to which people equate themselves from the external, separate from them. The paradoxical, and therefore contradictory, formula with identification is as follows: I = You.

Identifications are forms of adaptations to our external environment. In extreme cases, they are no more than subordinations and subjugations to other people and institutions that are more powerful than us. The powerful in turn like it when subordinates identify with their demands and believe that it is their own choice. That is why they encourage these identification processes as much as possible, through, for example family norms, religious rituals, corporate identity projects, financing of sporting events in which the athletes are presented as representatives of their nation etc.

In the public consciousness, identity is also frequently equated with social identity: I am = part of a bigger context (family, village, nation, religion...). The reverse conclusion is that I am nothing without being part of such a bigger system. This encourages a willingness to subjugate oneself to the demands of this greater unity, and to expect the same from others. This places external, rigid constraints on subjectivity and individuality. In an extreme case, our own interests have to be sacrificed in favour of the greater whole. This leads to the following paradox: in order to have an identity I have to give up my self. In exceptional circumstances, this can serve as the legitimation for perpetrators to act in the name of alleged higher principles and values.

These higher principles, which often only exist in the imagination or as purely legal structures, can suddenly vanish into thin air (for example because parents are getting divorced, because a company is being bought out by another company, or a state disappears after a lost war). Then those who previously identified themselves with 'family', 'company', or 'nation' cannot rely on anything specific to identify with, and are left with nothing.

Attributions

The second group of false assumptions over identity are types of attributions. By the attributions of other people or institutions, people are substantiated with characteristics to correspond with the others' goals and objectives. In dealing with attributions, the contradictory formula is as follows: You = I.

School grades or psychiatric diagnoses are examples of such forms of attributions. A school grade reveals nothing about the identity of the child, but rather ascribes him to a rank within a collective (his 'school class') in which he is compared to others ("He/she is a first class student"). A diagnosis like 'psychoses' or 'borderline personality disorder' does not reveal anything about the identity of the diagnosed person either. It merely discloses how psychiatric systems pigeonhole this person.

Attributions do not merely distribute characteristics amongst people, but they also express the expectations that have to be met from the viewpoint of the person who makes the attributions. For instance, a person receiving a psychiatric diagnosis must subordinate him- or herself to the psychiatric school of thought, and ideally take the prescribed medicine without question. Receiving the passport of a nation, a young man may need to enter military service, and failure to do so may quickly land him in prison.

Demarcations

A further serious fallacy regarding identity is to define one's identity by how we differ from others and how we differentiate ourselves from others, for example ...

- I am German and not a Turk!
- I do not want to be like my mother/ my father!
- I am a man and not a woman!
- I have to be the best!

With such efforts to differentiate ourselves (I ≠ You; I ≠ all of You) the external, the other or others, or the idea of the other or others, remains the point of reference rather than myself. If I differentiate myself from people with a particular nationality, or from 'refugees' or from 'asylum seekers' I still do not recognise who I really am. If you want to be different from your mother and father, you still take them as your benchmark for who you are, as your standard. A man still does not know how to behave as himself, even if he does not want to be a woman. Besides, which woman should he model himself on if there are so many women? To be better than others the person constantly has to keep his eye on the others so that they do not overtake him. He does not focus his attention on his own needs and skills but on other people. Competition blinds us to our own needs and constantly distracts us from ourselves.

In the same sense that conformity rarely leads to the development of one's own identity, and on the contrary is an expression of self-abandonment, nonconformism and the urge to be different or better than others also rarely leads to personal identity.

This "I am not like . . ." endeavour to create boundaries leads to distrust, envy, jealousy, greed, deception, and behaviour that lacks solidarity, and is essentially competitive. It lays bare all negative human traits. It constructs a front behind which we try to hide. We really want love and respect, but since we have been disappointed so often and deeply we no longer trust anyone. Our endeavour to create boundaries is an attempt to protect ourselves from further mental anguish.

For a long time I felt that I had to criticise the tenets of psychiatry, psychoanalysis, behavioural psychology, humanistic psychology, and systemic therapy, and even the tenets of trauma therapy, in order to validate my own theory. Every attempt resulted in the opposite. Since I started concentrating only on the development of my own theory and method I have inadvertently received encouragement and recognition. For me this means that I can certainly keep considering other psychological and psychotherapeutic concepts, and possibly learn something from their theoretical and practical errors.

True identity

In my view the identity formula is $I = I$. That is when there is actually something identical on both sides of the equal sign. What precisely does that mean? Human identity is the sum of all experiences the person has had since he or she was born, including the way he has reacted to these experiences and still manages them. This definition of identity takes into account the entire life biography of a person, and is receptive to further developments. Nobody is defined for the rest of his or her life, for example, by a particular 'diagnosis of illness' (i.e. schizophrenia). Every human is a system open to development.

Therefore, people are aware of their identity when they accept every experience they have had as truth and consciously remember it if necessary. That is easy with pleasant experiences whereas it is extremely difficult with traumatising experiences. Moreover, with unconsciously experienced traumatic incidents it is far more difficult than with conscious ones. Nevertheless, unconscious events are part of the human identity. They exist and are active in body and psyche. Traumatising events do not just disappear out of our living organism by themselves.

The time in our mother's womb, our birth, and the first two to three years of our life, we only store in a rudimentary way, not consciously. However, the recollection of that time we implicitly retain in our memory, and it can unconsciously influence our whole life, especially if we had traumatising experiences in these very early phases of life. (Ruppert, 2017; Wilks, 2017). Therefore, it is especially important to bring these early phases of life from the unconscious to the conscious mind.

To be

Through the fusion of a sperm and an egg cell, a new human life begins. A new person exists in the here and now, and wants to live and grow. For that, he or she is equipped with a flexible orientation plan, which is, as we know, contained in our genome. (Bauer, 2010). This new human being consists of matter, energy, and information, and already has a rudimentary psyche that grows alongside the rapidly developing body. Body and psyche constitute a single unit.

I consider the idea that the body of a child ('embryo') exists first before a 'soul' enters the body an error in reasoning. The separation of a living being into body and 'soul' does not make sense since the body needs a psyche to provide it with information, and navigate its needs right from the start. I consider this 'body' and 'soul' dualism a trauma survival strategy, because the main effect of traumatisation is that we try to minimise contact with our body, since we cannot bear the fear and pain which the body signals. The traumatised person is always present physically as well as in their psyche, even if he or she is not consciously aware of it.

I wanted to discover in one of my own resonance explorations how I had experienced the time in my mother's womb. It turned out that my first four weeks were a period of extreme uncertainty, and only later did it become evident that my mother had decided not to make any further attempt to abort me. I imagine it had to do with the fact that my parents had married quickly in both registry office and church as soon as my mother, who is a strict Catholic, realised she was pregnant. At least with the 'blessing of the church', I was allowed to exist.

Being the subject

Every newly formed human starts life as a subject and not just a mere thing ('object'). The unborn child has aims, and realises them by influencing his environment. That is how he convinces the maternal immune system not to see him as foreign protein, and so allow him to exist. He ensures through his own influence that there is a space for him in the uterus in which he can implant himself. Once there he allows the placenta to fuse with the womb and create an amniotic sac in which he can mature safely. The umbilical cord attaches him securely to the placenta and with that to the maternal organism.

A widespread trauma survival strategy is to deny that the unborn child has a psyche, presumably because then those involved in abortion do not have to feel incriminated. According to a statistic of the World Health Organisation every fourth pregnancy worldwide is terminated through human intervention, in other words the unborn child is killed (Hoppe, 2014).

To conduct an abortion, or to demand it (for example as the father of the child or the parents of the pregnant woman), means being an active perpetrator. Doctors and 'backstreet abortionists' who carry out an abortion are perpetrators. The woman who has an abortion i.e. who allows others to carry out an abortion on her is a perpetrator on the one hand, but also a trauma-victim on the other. Through the abortion emotional reactions of pain, grief, anger, disappointment, shame, and guilt emerge in her, which she cannot process consciously. Therefore, she has to block them out of her consciousness. Split off into her sub-consciousness, the feelings and memories of her abortion then take on a life of their own in her psyche.

Therefore, every abortion should be followed by psychotherapy so that the perpetrator-victim dynamic in the woman who has had the abortion does not become further reinforced and radicalised. The collaborators would also need therapeutic support to clarify their psyche and not to deny the act due to a sense of guilt and shame, then having to seek refuge in the position of a perpetrator.

When I was in my late twenties a girlfriend of mine became pregnant. Our relationship was turbulent, with a lot of cheating and phases of separation and reconciliation. This is why I did not resist when my girlfriend suggested that she should have an abortion. Our relationship afterwards did not last for very long, and we finally separated for good. When we met again after 11 years we both suddenly realised that our child would now be 11 years old, and as soon as we said this aloud we were both overcome by deep emotional pain.

We hugged and gave our tears free rein. This gave our relationship a much deeper level of closure, and we were both able to move on.

To be myself

The older the growing child becomes in the womb, the more she discovers herself. She realises her position in space, and can feel her skin, and can hear, smell and taste. Her brain matures allowing her to cope with increasingly complex sensor-motor tasks. Up until the date of birth more and more differentiated perceptions, movements, feelings, and cognitive achievements become possible (Chamberlain, 2010).

27

The unborn child increasingly recognises his mother. He communicates with her, tastes what she eats, smells her specific olfactory cues, listens to her voice, and prepares to look into her eyes as soon as he is born. He meets his mother with great attention and love even before birth, and counts on her love in return. For the unborn child it is existentially important not to feel isolated and alone while in the uterus. I have seen this in many therapeutic processes in which we have explored the client's prenatal time in depth.

What in psychiatry is diagnosed as 'depression', therefore, could stem from early experiences in the uterus. People affected with depression often see themselves in a black hole, into which they fall deeper and deeper, and from which they feel there is no escape. This conveys their experience when still an unborn child, in an infinite universe feeling completely abandoned and utterly alone in a uterus that rejects him.

Unfortunately, if a stable, healthy 'I' cannot develop in contact with the mother or father a healthy identity cannot develop either. Only fragmented memories remain, and important aspects of one's biography fade from memory. This makes it impossible to foster one's personal happiness internally. One becomes incapable of paying sufficient attention to oneself to be able to create healthy relationships, in which each participant gains an advantage and a zest for life from the other. Without my own 'I', I am unpredictable as a person for myself and for others.

Healthy, stressed, and traumatised psyche

Roughly classified our human psyche can find itself in three states:

- *Healthy state:* Here we are open for everything that shows itself in objective reality (level 1), and for what is present within ourselves (level 2 reality). The prerequisite for this is that we feel safe. This makes us curious about anything else in the world: nature, people, things, technology etc. In this inner calm and unstrained state, there is plenty of room for feelings such as love and happiness. The whole organism is well demarcated from the environment, and at the same time open to it. In situations of conflict, we remain calm and look for a suitable and effective long-term solution for all concerned.

- *Stressful state:* If we feel threatened, our psyche switches to stress mode. Perception, feelings, ideas, and thinking concentrate on the danger. Fear, anger, and rage are the prevailing feelings in stress mode producing aggressive ideas, thoughts, and actions. In a conflict situation we choose short-term, and often violent, solutions. We remain in this mode until the perceived danger is over. Only then can the psyche return to its healthy and relaxed mode described above.

- *Traumatic state:* If we cannot cope with the danger and our stress mode actions fail to resolve the situation, but on the contrary make it even worse and more hopeless, the psychological emergency mode has to suppress the stress state and switch it off. It is no longer useful, but instead is a disadvantage to us. That is when the trauma-emergency-mechanism comes into play. This allows us to hide and deny the threatening reality as much as possible. We reduce our perceptions, become weak and emotionally numb, and no longer think clearly. We dissociate ourselves from our experience, and are unable to remember consciously and clearly what we experienced at the time. Our psyche falls into a state in fundamental contradiction to its existential purpose of trying to access reality as it really is. In its attempt to misinterpret reality rather than recognising it as it is, the psyche has to sacrifice its unity and cohesion; one part continues to capture reality as it is, and the other part does not. The part that renounces reality breaks free of its connection to the body as much as possible ('dissociation'); it goes 'into the head' (reality level 3). In my experience, this fundamental split between wanting to recognise reality and having to deny it constitutes the basis for most psychological abnormalities and physical signs of illness.

The boundaries of self-awareness

The human psyche is well designed to serve human beings. This is why it specialises in average size dimensions and time lapses. As humans, we do not instantly notice things that are too big, too small, too fast, too slow, too 'ethereal', or too dense. There is a tremendous diversity of objectively existing realities of which we are not aware, but which we can only tap into to some extent through our thinking ability.

As an instrument for the recognition of reality, the human psyche finds it difficult to understand itself when it is in the process of this recognition. People barely notice the activities of their psyche. They struggle to understand the reality and the operating principle of their psyche, or at least to accept it. This is why some people go as far as to deny that the psyche exists at all and that it could be important and meaningful. Their belief is that everything humans do is the result of physical and chemical processes, and therefore determined purely by matter. Neurosciences are currently fashionable and easily promote neurobiologism; recently a student in one of my lectures claimed that the experience of love is merely down to certain hormones in the brain.

It is much easier to recognise the many dimensions of the psyche in other people than in ourselves. This is why we are more likely to detect psychological defects in others than in ourselves. We see how foolish, crazy, and obstinate other people can be, yet barely recognise our own ignorance and confusion.

Competition and shame also cloud our self-awareness. Someone who gives the impression of being psychologically impaired or even 'sick' is quickly shunned and socially ostracized. At job interviews a 'psychological diagnosis' generally guarantees a failure to secure the position. The aim of a competitive society, therefore, is to appear as intelligent and rational as possible, so people conceal defects in their psyche and hide psychological errors of performance or judgement, even from themselves. Everybody wants to appear as 'smart' and 'intelligent' as possible. Amongst young people, this is considered to be 'cool'. And this, for example, is how a senior manager can play the rational, clever decision-maker during the day, and at night visit his 'domina' and ask and allow her to humiliate him like a helpless child.

The illusion of psychological health

As long as almost everybody participates in this game of deception, it works to the motto: "If you spare me from having to declare my psychological defects I will not reveal what I notice about you either." Moreover, the more authority and power someone holds, the less the people dependent on him or her dare to voice that which is obvious: this person has a deep psychological defect and is in desperate need of psychotherapy!

The invisible per se, and the psyche's conscious effort to render something invisible, cause widespread ignorance of reality. For instance, most believe that it is enough to reset a splintered bone after a traffic accident; the fact that the splintered psyche after an accident also needs to be reset remains outside general awareness (Sauer and Emmerich, 2017). The fragmented body parts may heal, but parts of the psyche may remain at the accident scene, and still feel and perceive as if the accident had only just happened. The same applies for a traumatising childbirth, when the child is separated from her mother and put into baby ward. The human psyche and the damages inflicted on it receive little attention in society (Ahrens-Eipper & Nelius, 2017).

To generally believe that one's psyche is healthy is an enormous illusion. To have the healthiest possible psyche at our disposal for our own life we have to take care of it accordingly. The psyche is extremely sensitive and prone to failure. It may have compensative and repair mechanisms at its disposal (for example, it regenerates while we are sleeping), nevertheless there are many demanding situations in life with which the individual psyche cannot cope. This particularly holds true in the early developmental stages; the younger we are, the easier it is for our psyche to be traumatised.

We are better off assuming the possibility that our psyche does not function very well, and may even be traumatised, than to think that everything is in good working order as it is. On the other hand, it is important for me to emphasise that even if 100% of people in society have a traumatised psyche, the same 100% of people still have healthy psychic structures that they can rely on. Nobody should feel ashamed of having been the victim of a traumatising experience in life. No child is guilty because she was severely psychologically injured. The more people in society who openly admit to having had psychotraumatic experiences, the easier it will be for others to be open and honest with themselves as well.

Hardware and Software

The psyche is more complex and contradictory than our everyday understanding so far is able to grasp. Why, for example, are people curious about life on other planets, and yet at the same time at a breakneck speed destroy the diversity of life on our own planet? Why do people search for the origins of the universe, and yet show little interest in exploring their own personal history? Why do most people consider themselves to be good and friendly, and yet continue to agree to the use of military force, or violence in the raising of children?

In the western nations, the widespread opinion prevails that we cope well with 'psychological disturbances' by the means of psychiatry and psychoactive drugs, and that we are close to developing further suitable medicines or genetic solutions. That is a big self-deception. We have to face up to the truth that we must engage with ourselves in a much deeper and more intensive way in order not to become a prisoner of our own psyche. It is a serious logical error to equate our psyche with our brain and other physical metabolic processes. Brain and body merely supply the hardware that allows the running of many psychological 'software-programs'. As is shown in the research of so-called 'multiple personality disorders', numerous personality-programs can run simultaneously and in parallel in a human organism (Huber, 2011).

As interesting as these neuroscientific research results are, at the end of the day they do not help us any further in understanding our psyche. In the same sense, in the computer industry no engineer or technician would seriously claim to understand computer software, or even to be able to reprogram a computer, simply through studying computer hardware.

Preservation of the species or the self?

The main purpose of the psyche is to preserve the living organism on the one hand, and the species on the other. For that, we have feelings of hunger and thirst, sexual desire and needs, as well as empathy and love for children and feelings of extreme grief and pain when our own children, partner, or close relatives are in distress, or dying.

However, in this we also find contradictions. The survival of the individual organism can suffer *for* the survival of the species, or conversely the survival of the person can be in the way of the survival of the species. Wanting children raises the question of how much of your vital energy, time, and resources will you have to provide, or even sacrifice, for your children. In societies based on monetary systems this simply means: How much will having children cost me? How many children can I actually afford financially? At least men often think that way if it depends on them being able to come up with the necessary funds to support the family. However, even women can be ripped out of their dreams of having children if after a divorce they suddenly become a 'single parent' and may have to rely on social welfare.

So children are always in danger of abandonment, parental abuse or neglect when they get in the way of their parents' desire for self-preservation. The evil stepmother, who favours her own children and rejects the children of the other woman, is not just a fairy tale, but bitter reality for many children.

3
Psyche and Society

Psychological knowledge is important for all of us

Thus, we do need a sound and critical examination of our own psyche. Unfortunately, in some places psychology is an academic subject that trains inquisitive students to become academics, far removed from real life. In my opinion, a significant misconception about psychology taught at universities is the idea that everyone is responsible for their own problems. It is as though it is merely a question of attitudes, stance, and 'resilience' as to whether someone is doing well psychologically or not. Everything that inflicts traumatic damage from the outside is blanked out or dismissed as trivial. Moreover, psychology in traumatised societies is abused so as to intimidate, manipulate, control, lie to, and terrorise individuals or groups of people. For example, advertising agencies offer psychological services to the military and intelligence services so that they can create propaganda images of an enemy as a preparation for war, and convince the public that it is worthwhile to kill other human beings (Mausfeld, 2017).

Whereas I consider it a crucial task for those of us who are professional psychologists to develop knowledge of the human psyche so as to help all, including those without an academic education, better understand who they really are. Everyone urgently needs to know what problems the psyche can have and cause, and how he/she can improve with the help of his/her psyche, so that everyone, in his own way, can contribute to the prevention of psychotrauma and the development of more constructive and less damaging relationships and societies.

Nobody should allow themselves to be dominated by the inner conflicts and trauma-survival strategies of others, and thereby have to permanently forfeit happiness in their own life.

If we want to develop together for the better, we must not just delegate knowledge about our own psyche to 'experts', politicians, founders of religion or pastoral workers, doctors, or psychologists. Indeed, the fixation on 'leaders', 'gurus', 'heroes', or 'shamans' is yet another trauma-survival strategy of people who had to give up on their own 'I', and now instead search for their happiness through identification with someone else, in the doctrine of salvation. Everyone has to be able to become the expert on his own psyche! Everyone has to assume responsibility for his psyche, understand why he is the way he is, and understand why others act the way they do. If we regard ourselves with indifference, we will consider other people with indifference too.

The need for an enlightening psychology for everyone is one of the reasons why I do not value or give much importance to academic degrees or titles in the trainings that I offer. Everyone who is prepared to confront himself with his life biography can become a good psychologist; it is not necessary to have written a doctoral thesis. Only those who dare to confront themselves with their own traumata can provide helpful support for others on their path of self-discovery in an optimal way.

'Psychological disorders' not only have an impact on the health and happiness of every individual; as we know by now parents inevitably transfer their psychological problems onto their children through the bonding process. Psychological traumas work across generations. Parents offload their traumas onto their children, and the children, in their primal love for their parents, try to take on the psychological burdens of their parents. Therefore children connect unconsciously with the traumatic experiences of their parents, and sometimes even of their grandparents (Baer & Frick-Baer, 2010, Ruppert, 2012). Even if children fight externally, and reject their parents, always behind is the child's unappeased longing for the love of their mum and dad. This leads to disastrous and unresolvable entanglements between parents and children. Both sides can neither bond together nor separate in a good way. Traumatised parents cannot leave their children alone, and the children unconsciously remain fixated on their mothers and fathers for their entire life. From a psychological perspective then, the children never really mature and become autonomous.

Since families and parent-child relationships are at the core of every society this has consequences that go far beyond the family; when psychologically traumatised children become adults they carry their psychological disturbances into all areas of society: education, employment, and political systems. A substantial part of the psyche remains caught in the unpleasant childhood. Because of their childhood traumatisation, they are not able to perceive, feel, and think actual realities at all but only their distorted versions of reality. They construct their own world, following their illusions and invented principles that often are contrary to reality, and so they remain stuck in the illusory world of their childlike trauma-survival strategies.

In this way many expect to finally get the love that they never received from their parents from a spouse or friends, but at the same time the damaged parts of their psyche cannot allow true intimacy, because that would remind them of the primal traumas of their childhood and be much too painful. Instead, the spouse has to be kept at a safe distance so as not to activate the old pains and fears. Arguments about unimportant issues are commonplace in relationships.

Seemingly adult people can make demands on the economic and work systems just like immature children, wanting everything immediately. Others gamble on the stock market as though it was just another kind of computer game, or allow their intelligence and creativity to be exploited for the profit of an employer in the production of things that are harmful to others. Some live in a small world of never-ending thirst for acceptance and attention, stuck in their earlier damaged psyche.

Still others transfer their self-denial, learned in childhood, onto the economic system and their place of work, making no demands, allowing themselves to be fobbed off with low wages and cheap words of thanks. Just as with their own parents, they cannot say no to the demands of superiors and colleagues, and voluntarily take on so much work that eventually they buckle under the strain and suffer from 'burnout' in the end.

The latter would have probably happened to me, too, if I had not started at around 40 years old to realise my psychotrauma and gradually wake up from my illusions. In groups, I was quick to say yes when there was something to do. I was always focused on the external and ready to meet the expectations of others. For a while, I also thought I should engage in party politics and so for a few years I was a member of the newly established Green Party in Germany. However, I was always secretly hoping to be respected and noticed by other people for my engagement.

For some early traumatised people politics are an opportunity to try to overcome the helplessness of their childhood. Unconsciously split off feelings of fear, anger, grief, and humiliation are the engine for touching the machinations of power and the desire to make changes in society. In accordance with their childhood survival-strategies they are searching in the field of politics for options, for example, to redirect their hatred and anger for their parents towards certain groups in society ('foreigners', 'asylum seekers'...). Some are so hardened internally that they will drag the whole of society (i.e. their parents) into the abyss with them. When they come to power they handle tanks, guns and bombs with bravado and noise, as though they were participants in some enormous game of adventure between small, adolescent boys.

Due to their traumatisation, many in the field of politics like to appear as if they know everything and they behave arrogantly. Others are financed by those who help them gain power without any critical attention to the particular interests involved. Still others try to save society from ruin, standing up for the poor and weak, and caring about social justice, just as they had to care about and save their traumatised parents, or protect their siblings from their parents' violence as children. Strategies of violence are more often the choice of men in politics, whereas strategies of balance and harmony are more often the specialtity of women.

Even when politicians are elected to office in democracies, it is not guaranteed that they focus on the interests of their voters. They often try to disguise their own ideas of 'economy', 'social issues', or 'inner security' with slogans that help them to win. What they do after their election is down to them, since there is no obligation to actually fulfil promises in a representative democracy. The real policies the powerful of one's party decide according to the relevant financial and economic situation and the military balance of power on the international stage (Mausfeld, 2017).

The traumatised voters act accordingly, putting themselves into the position of dependent children who make demands of their parents, fully aware that the final say is with the parents who make the decisions. Some politicians then find themselves on the receiving end of the contempt, anger, and hatred that some people could not express towards their own traumatising parents. Some voters subject themselves blindly and with admiration to 'their' president, chancellor, or minister. Neither the politician nor the 'electorate' are even vaguely aware of these unconscious dynamics permeated by trauma.

Are Parents for or against children?

We humans are social creatures, and we need other humans for our life and our development. We existentially depend on other people. This starts with our conception. The developing child needs the organism of his mother, in which he can grow and, after nine months, be born. He needs his mother and her body for at least three more years so that his psyche can stabilise and be steady. The child is reliant on a caring and loving mother at all costs. Consequently being a mother of small children is a fulltime job that no one can manage as a sideline. The notion of a 'compatibility' between family and a time-intensive career is an illusion, or rather a societal dogma that operates at the expense of both mothers and children.

For a healthy psychological and physical development, the child also needs the support of her father. In her environment, she needs many people who offer loving and friendly encounters, giving examples of a good and constructive coexistences.

Unfortunately, this is not always the situation. Many children are unwanted and not loved by their parents. Many children are conceived and born into social conditions which confront them with rejection, hostility, and threat. The child has no power in such situations, and if she wants to live she has to make herself useful to others, this becoming the only means by which she can survive. When the pros and cons of having children are considered in Germany the argument is often raised that children are necessary to safeguard pensions.

Many traumatised parents are unable to act in the interest of their children. They place their own trauma-survival interests above the needs of their children, and abuse their children for their survival needs. In this way, countless children become victims of their traumatised mothers and/or fathers. The child's parents become his first trauma-perpetrators. The American psycho-historian Lloyd de Mause has got to the heart of this worldwide situation for children in his book The History of Childhood: Untold Story of Child Abuse: 'The history of childhood is a nightmare, from which we are only just waking up.' (de Mause, 1980)

Mothers and fathers that cannot cope with their own life will cling onto their children as their saviours, and do not leave them in peace. They disguise their own trauma-survival strategies as 'care' and 'help' for their children.

The absence of maternal affection

The relationship with our mother is the first and most funda-mental societal relationship. In my experience, it shapes the basic attitude to all further and later societal relationships.

Hans-Joachim Maaz (2017) gives a striking account of how a missing or misunderstood mothering lays the cornerstone for the lifelong inner plight of humans. He also points out how social circumstances are ruined if a healthy mothering is missing in a society. The essential guarantor for a healthy physical and psychological development of the child lies in being welcomed by his or her mother, her loving attention and her willingness to protect her child from anything that could hurt him physically or mentally.

Therefore, a woman must be not just physically able and ready to become a mother, she needs to be psychologically capable of giving the child time and space in her body and in her life. Nobody should persuade or force women to have children. First, a woman has to remove all obstacles that block her, not just in a biological, but also in a psychological sense, in order to become a mother. This includes her own traumatising experiences as an unborn child, at her birth, after birth, as an infant and toddler, of not having been wanted, loved, or protected by her own mother and her father (Ruppert, 2014). Being a mother only succeeds based on free will and confrontation of her ambivalence, in face of the considerable restriction to her independence temporarily for the benefit of the child. She has to make her body and her psyche fully available for this other living being for at least three years. Those who do not see the joy in this or the benefit for their own growth should seriously consider if they really want to become mothers.

The same holds true for men who want to become fathers. To have a child means biologically being the father, but being a father is much more than that. It is the effort to offer the child loving contact, to provide protection, and pave the way to a healthy autonomy for the child. For many children the lack of a mother unfortunately continues with the lack of a father as well.

Education for or against children?

Many see 'education' of children generally as necessary in order to turn them into capable adults. According to Freudian psychoanalysis the child – a creature of instinct – has to be 'socialised' through the development of a super ego, in other words through the imposition of cultural norms and rules. On the one hand, the question arises as to whether children are in fact antisocial by nature; on the other we have to consider what kind of adults children become when raised by these norms and prohibitions. And how do these norms and prohibitions even present themselves? For whose benefit are they, and to whose detriment? And what is the effect on children if their upbringing is primarily focused in them being better and more successful than their peers? Do they really become social beings, or instead do they turn into inconsiderate 'peak performers' who do not care who pays the price for their personal success?

Thus the traumatisation of children by their traumatised parents continues during their 'education', with children seen as objects of reward and punishment. Without proper reflection, educators and teachers will transmit their own good and bad childhood experiences onto the children. Alice Miller (2006) describes this as 'black pedagogy'.

In most societies parents are seen as naturally competent, and as doing right by their children. Even when studying teaching methods, students are not required to have a look at their own childhood traumas before accompanying children on their journey into the world. This is why perpetrator-victim-dynamics between nannies and children and teachers and children are generally the order of the day worldwide.

I attended a small village school for my first four school years, which had a lower room for classes 1 to 3 and an upper room for classes 4 to 8. There I had to deal with a relatively nice subordinated lady teacher, but also with a male teacher who, despite his violence to us children, was promoted to a 'Superior Teacher'. All the children feared this man since he brutally slapped children in the face, sending some children flying to the floor. With terror, I still remember the image of one of my classmates nearly having his ear ripped off as he was pulled off the school bench. To make these blows particularly painful he would turn the heavy ring on his finger around. Hitting us with a ruler or a long pointed stick was relatively harmless compared to this.

He had a prosthesis for his lower left arm, apparently caused by a war wound, the cause of which we children never heard anything, whereas every day we did have to hear his bellowing which pierced through the walls from the upper classroom to the lower. His shouting would get worse when military aircraft raced across the sky. I was never sure if he was for or against the war:

an old Nazi or a new democrat. One thing was for sure: he led his own war against us children every day in the classroom or in the schoolyard.

Rivalry between men and women

Another kind of dependency relationship that can end in perpetrator-victim-dynamics we can see in the relationships of one sex to another. Sexuality as a form of reproduction with two genders serves the survival of the human species. Therefore, men and women depend on each other for the purpose of reproduction, and for that, they have to be in contact with each other. Concerning their sexual function, however, they have very different needs and perceptions of their natural and social environment. For men sexual relations with a woman can be a one-off act in order to become the father of a child. For women procreation completely changes their life. Once she is pregnant a woman has to endure the 9-month process of pregnancy, a risky birth process and, after giving birth, she is responsible for the child for many years.

Whether the father provides helpful support with any of these responsibilities remains to be seen. By the existence of the child, men in a sense lose 'their' woman, particularly emotionally, to the child. She is often no longer available as sexual partner to the same extent as before, and many husbands may become sexually frustrated and may even demand sex by violence and pressure. Many married men may have the tendency to enter extramarital affairs, seek prostitutes, or find another, often younger, partner.

It is the case that men generally want sexual intercourse significantly more often than women do, within and outside of the partnership. Sigmund Freud saw in the male libido a primeval need: every man wants to have sex with as many women as possible and therefore constantly rivals other men. Looking at the kings of the former Ottoman Empire with their harems of women, or today looking at Africa, for example Swaziland, where the king is allowed to have sex with all young women on his territory, seem to support Freud's thinking. Some men act as animals do: "I am the strongest, the best looking ... and I have the biggest penis! And I want sex all the time! That is why the most beautiful women belong to me! No other man is allowed to touch them! Or else I become aggressive!"

In turn, many women behave like their evolutionary predecessors: in the fight between men, they wait and see who wins the upper hand and then take the winner for sexual intercourse. Biologists call it the 'Ladies' choice' (Miersch, 2002, p. 63ff). In return, women often expect material gifts and financial provision for their sexual favours. Still, infidelity is not alien to women either. If someone comes along and flirts with her, and appears physically more attractive than her now a little aged partner, she may not categorically say no.

Sexuality is a source of lust and pleasure. However it can also become one of the biggest potentials for stress in the lives of men and women, if infidelity, jealousy and abandonment occur: "Since my husband went to another family a year ago I am completely beside myself. We had just married – after a two-year relationship. Immediately before he left our daughter and me we had bought a house at his request and we had renovated it ourselves. After we moved in, he even built a garden pond and ordered new furniture. Then suddenly he became incredibly aggressive towards me and shortly after he told me that he intended to go on holiday with another woman and that everything is over!" (Excerpt from an email message to me)

Sexuality can also be traumatising...

- if sex is forced with violence or in return for money,
- if pregnancies and births are traumatising events for women and...
- if children are forced to satisfy the sexual needs of adults.

Besides sex, men and women are also searching for intimacy, love and comfort, they want material and emotional security from someone of the opposite gender; in the case of same-sex couples, these same needs hold true. This can lead to some making an exclusive claim of ownership of their partner: "You belong to me! I watch jealously that nobody else comes close to you, and you do not give your love to anyone else!"

With the state of being 'in love', which is an exceptional high hormonal situation, the notion that "you are the only one!" is used by both as a statement of their special love. However, when this exceptional state fades, because familiarisation returns the hormones to their normal levels, this 'being in love' state may be experienced as annoying and restricting of one's autonomy, even to the point that we want to separate from the other. This is why it frequently happens that one partner wants to continue the relationship while the other does not. One tries to pull away, and the other clings. The process of separation becomes particularly conflicted if they have children, and joint material assets have been accumulated which are difficult to divide equally.

It seems that the enormous potential for love that humans have at their disposal is as great as the potential for aggression, which can be activated in close relationships. If we are scared of being rejected and let down by the person who is the focus of our sexual desire and love, many of us completely lose our composure.

The more stressed we become, the more our disappointment and frustration build up to hatred and aggression, and so many partnerships are a breeding ground for physical and verbal abuse and violence.

Any decrease in sexual attraction lowers the tolerance threshold for the 'disruptive' behaviours and attitudes of the partner further. Disappointed expectations of love, and hurt pride turn former loving affairs into battlefields of physical and psychological cruelties. Occasionally it becomes a life-long mission for the disappointed partner to ruin their companion emotionally, financially, and physically.

The fights of the sexes, and corresponding attempts to bring this into some kind of bearable form through cultural, social, and legal regulations has existed since the beginning of mankind. One look at reality shows that many people become the trauma victim of their once beloved partner, and by defending them-selves they, too, become trauma-perpetrators.

At just six years old I was head-over-heels in love with a neigh-bourhood girl two doors down the road from me. For a long time she remained my reference point for the unattainable woman, even though I had one or two girlfriends when I was in puberty. My fixation on that girl, which I now know signified a trauma-survival-strategy for the lack of connection with my mother, was further complicated in my puberty by sexual fixations. I scanned every woman as a possible sexual partner, and this made me reflect on how I needed to be as a man in order for a woman to like and admire me. I did not see my true self, but rather saw myself through the eyes of women and their needs.

My parents (born 1933 and 1934 respectively) had warned me not to 'knock up' a woman, because that would inevitably mean I would have to marry. However, with this warning they unwittingly revealed their own story, of which they never talked. However, when I calculated my own birth I realised my mother must have been at least one month pregnant when she got married – in white. In those days, and in a strictly catholic village, a 'white wedding' was only allowed if the bride was a virgin. My mother's oldest brother also had made a refugee woman pregnant right after the war, and had to get married quickly. The birth control pill only became available in Germany from the 1960s onwards.

Nobody knew how to handle shame in our family. We suppressed and separated it off, but repeatedly found some pleasure in the shaming of others, and in an exaggerated display of pride.

Economic competition

For us humans it is difficult to achieve a good life just through our own work. We are reliant on others who use the land and natural resources as well. Therefore, we are reliant on coopera-tion, division of labour, and amicable solutions to conflicts in our striving for property and land, means of food and material production, and welfare. Work is not just a necessity; it can provide help with our self-development. Joachim Bauer describes this as follows "Even the self-sustaining, need-satisfying effects of working are a part of this encounter with the self, just as much as the contribution to our personal identity through experiences and competencies gained by working. After all, work also always means an encounter with others, with our social environment". (Bauer, 2013, S. 15)

Strangely enough in most societies today, it is an unquestioned dogma that competition and rivalry are unavoidable, and not an expression of insufficiently developed humanity, but rather that they are urgently needed in order to achieve a functioning economy and division of labour. Since Adam Smith, the constantly invoked 'invisible hand' of market development is meant to ensure that in an ideally unregulated 'competition of producers' goods, allegedly always 'in short supply', get to the consumer at the right price. Moreover, due to 'shortage' a continuous and never-ending 'increase' is the presupposition for everything to function for the good of society.

Rivalry instead of cooperation supports the common good? More and more is required and the work has to be done faster and faster, so that everyone can live a satisfying life? Does the wealth of the affluent automatically 'trickle down' to the poor? These are absurd ideas! Especially where the most appropriate production of vital necessities and their distribution is at play (i.e. for housing, food, clean water, and appropriate clothing). It seems that we take the animalistic algorithm of sexual rivalry between men and women, and childish envy, as the bases for an entire economic framework.

So, the disadvantages of economic competition and blind expectations of growth are obvious: envy, frustration, aggression, malicious joy, conflict, and discord are the order of the day. Winners and losers emerge from a competitive economic system, what the one has the other would like to have too. If one person has found a lucrative way to generate income, another tries to do the same thing and snatch away customers and 'markets'.

If someone wins, another loses. Moreover, it is even tougher than that: I have to make sure the other fails so that I keep winning and do not become a 'loser' myself. There are always losers in a system based on competition, both with employers as well as those who earn a living by their labour. The failure of businesses and the unemployment of wage earners are two sides of the same coin. Working in such a system means being permanently under stress and threatened by professional 'burn-out'. Those without work and earning potential are equally stressed and have the tendency to become depressed. So work is a source of stupidity and meaninglessness.

In the competition of business those who are 'losers' are also exhausting material, financial, and psychological resources with the benefit for no one. In a single stroke a competitor's innovation, a financial bubble or a stock market crash can destroy everything that has been developed with great effort and expense over many years. People lose their jobs, companies move abroad, and once thriving cities become deserted.

'Economy', in the true sense of the word, actually means a careful budgeting with the available resources for a good life. Economic competition, however, leads to wastage of materials, time, and money on the one hand, and to shortages, poverty, disappointment and boredom on the other. One side's profit results in the other side's poverty. The financial profit of some is the financial debt of others (Graeber, 2014). Empirically, the gap between winners and losers then widens. It is no secret, that the eight richest men in the world own more capital than is available to the poorer half of the world population Consequently, over time there will be more and more poor people, and fewer and fewer rich ones in a 'system of competition'. In the end a handful of large corporations control all market development and impose their own ideas and interests on society. They enjoy complete freedom whilst the 'losers' are subjected to the daily pressure of making money and paying off their debts.

Such an economic system is chronically unstable because of its 'competition' and the eternal 'push for growth'. Predictably and with regularity, it comes to bankruptcies, collapses, inflations, unemployment, and social unrest (Senf, 2005). The rivalry for employment, natural resources, and means of production by necessity can lead to armed conflicts. Whoever has the best weapons can steal land, people, natural resources, and trading routes. The last 200 years, during which capitalism and imperialism have gone hand in hand, have shown that the 'invisible hand of the market' would not survive for one day without the visible fist of the military and police forces, since it creates too many conflicts of interest. Thus, perpetrator-victim dynamics are common in a competitive economy.

Fighting tooth and nail in competitive business does not concern competitors, and within such organisations envy, resentment, and mobbing and scheming reign. A nerve-wracking psychological war goes on for higher wages and better jobs, and nobody can really trust anyone else in a competitive economy. Today's friend may be tomorrow's archrival. If someone is too open and admits their mistakes, he or she may soon learn how easily an opponent can threaten their position.

There is no long-term security in a competitive economy, neither for the companies nor for the working people. In a situation where abstract values such as money and profit are the measure for all economic activity, people live like slaves for such an economy, sometimes working themselves to death. They work against each other, instead of working together and laying the foundations for a good life.

The fixation on profits and the fear of loss of employment hinders independent and critical perception, feeling and thinking in all parties. People have to subjugate all of their mental capacity to monetary increases. Money is not a means to leading a good life, but everybody serves with his or her psyche a monetary system that does not care about the way in which profits are reached. What brings in money and contributes to monetary increase seems 'reasonable' and 'rational'. The striving to get money in order to make more money becomes an overarching end in itself. The resulting indifference concerning real products is how this economy mirrors the indifference towards the people participating in this type of economy. Only those who have money and capital, or who make their labour available as cheaply as possible are of interest. In many regions of Germany refugees are seen as particularly interesting since they remedy the labour shortage. Those who are not willing to work for a pittance are not interesting and redundant. Compassion for the victims of this kind of economy is readily dismissed as 'sentimental' and left to the private initiatives of 'do-gooders' and the welfare state.

Since competition means ruthlessness and selfishness, this also influences how we handle natural resources in a competitive economy, the principle being to gain as much profit as possible from environmental destruction. Winnings are a private matter. The removal of the damage is a public responsibility. "How smart would it be then, if astronauts were to poison the oxygen supply of their spaceship? Yet that is exactly what humanity is doing. And has been doing for over 300 years, since market societies made an appearance, in which exchange value has won against quality of life and profit has gained the sole, absolute power over human psyche and actions." (Varoufakis, 2015, p. 126).

Through schooling and the education system, the idea of competition and 'achievement' is implanted early into the minds of children and young adults, even against their will (Kohn, 1989). Those with worse grades than others have no prospect of getting the better-paid jobs. Cooperation becomes a luxury that no pupil or student can afford to indulge in, and envy, resentment, and shame are widespread amongst students, so they are well prepared for the fierce competition that is waiting for them in their working life.

In my school days, I suffered a lot under this competitive system. When I got bad grades I was shamed in front of my teachers and parents, especially since good grades for me were a rare means of receiving some little favourable attention from my parents. That is also how I got my first admonition in high school, which I was deeply ashamed about, because I had forged my father's signature on a very poor school grade, so amateurishly done that even my short-sighted Latin teacher noticed it.

However, if my grades were good my peers teased me. When I constantly had better grades than my classmates, I was called a 'geek' and excluded from certain friendship cliques. So the only choice offered to me by this school system was between nuisance and pariah, and I increasingly became a lone wolf who trusted nobody.

Political and national rivalry

For the healthy development of children, for lasting partnerships and good parenthood, and for stable forms of economic division of labour a superordinate social frame is needed which strives to enable everybody to have a good life. It would require a political system that specifies a legal framework that is clear and valid for all, and to which all concerned can contribute in decisions for the common good. In particular, the community needs protection from the ruthlessness and violence of some individuals. The interests of individual members should not harm the community as a whole.

Political systems define themselves in the first place through the territorial area in which their legislation is valid. Historically we can see that we have developed from initially small family clan structures into monarchical form of rule (dukedoms, principalities, kingdoms, empires) and on to the nation states of today. Currently in 2018, there are 193 nation states that are members of the United Nations. In addition, there is the Vatican City and 12 territories whose state property is contested, or which are in free association with other states.

The guiding principle of nation states is, analogous to the largely predominant competing economy, one of inter-nation competition. The closer that states border alongside each other, the more competitive they are, and the larger their conflicts of interest can become, for example, when there are mutual demands on the territory of another country, and its natural and human resources are opened up. Therefore, the issue of war is always on the agenda between nation states. As a result, all nation states equip themselves with arms that are intended to protect the state authority from attacks by other states and, if necessary, enable the invasion of other states. To avoid this they enter into political alliances of convenience and declare their aims as 'national defence', for the preservation of legitimate, national interests. As part of this all national states have additional secret services that interfere with the internal affairs of other states, commit acts of terrorism, instigate riots, eliminate political opponents, conduct secret warfare, beyond democratic parliaments and elected politicians (Ganser, 2016a).

The claims of a nation state, not just on its own population and natural resources, but also on those of other states, can be not just regional, but are also general and global, and they lead to colonialism and imperialism. Repeatedly in the course of human history, nation states have tried to subject other states and communities under their power. Amongst others the Greeks, the Persians, the Huns, the Vikings, the Romans, the various African Kingdoms, the Maya, the Inca, the Chinese, the Ottomans, the Turks, the Portuguese, the Spanish, the British, the French, the Germans, and the Japanese have all tried with more or less success, incurring the large scale distribution of fear, disease, and death. Essentially human history is nothing more than a bleak accumulation of conquests, pillages, raids, and enslavements.

Currently there is one particular nation, the United States of America, which pursues global imperial aims and is capable of practically enforcing them with the use of its military might to invade other countries. Through its so called 'intelligence services' and its support of terror organisations, it stages, openly or secretly, the overthrow of a government and supports the change of leadership, if it is in its interests. Greece, Spain, Italy, Iran, Korea, Vietnam, Panama, Honduras, Chile, Turkey, Nicaragua, Afghanistan, Iraq, Ukraine, Lybia, Syria, Venezuela – the list of overt and covert American wars against other countries and the construction of dictatorships in many of those countries after the end of the Second World War is alarmingly long (Ganser, 2016b). Unfortunately, this list is still not finished. Currently, only the USA has the necessary military and economic means to implement its ambitions towards world supremacy directly.

Only Russia can seriously curb the imperial claims of the US, since that state did not just emerge as a victorious power after WWII, but also has at its disposal a large nuclear armament and enough of its own energy reserves and natural resources. Currently only Russia can plausibly threaten the United States of America with a prolonged war, or even total annihilation, by atomic bombs.

Therefore, the Third World War is already happening, and has done so since the end of the WWII, as a proxy war between America and Russia (Lüders, 2015). WW III is yet undecided, even if the United States currently does have many more weapons, military bases and global influence than Russia. However the USA have decided what ideological system should prevail, in a dispute that has dominated politics in the 20th century – 'capitalism' or 'communism' – in America's favour. Meanwhile, the alleged human right to global exploitation and individual mega-riches is enforced everywhere, and seems to most people living today a natural law that nobody can change.

Communism as a political system and guiding principle has practically ceased to exist after the self-dissolution of the Soviet Union – with one small exception: North Korea. Even here, though, the United States tries to scare this country through economic sanctions and military threats. Foolishly, North Korea's ally is mighty China, and by now, it has some nuclear warheads with matching long-range missiles and a political leadership which fancies itself in a war of David versus Goliath. At this time (since autumn 2017) the world is a step closer to the total abyss of nuclear destruction.

Otherwise, all remaining states have subordinated themselves to the capitalistic claim to world supremacy of the USA. Even the People's Republic of China is only a communist form of governance on a political level. On an economic level this densely populated country practices an uninhibited capitalistic competitiveness that now puts the fear of losing even into the USA, who were so used to winning.

What ignites political conflicts most at the moment is the fight for raw materials, and most of all for fossil fuels such as crude oil and natural gas. That is why at present there is the war in Syria. That is why the Middle East is and has been the focal point of many international political conflicts and illegal wars since the end of the Second World War. All of which are in conflict with the rules of the United Nations that no nation states should forcibly interfere with the internal affairs of other states and attack them militarily, but rather should respect their sovereignty (Ganser, 2016 b and c). Nevertheless, the UN is not a democratic institution; what really counts is the strength of those states with the greatest military power.

Natural disasters would suffice

Earth is a burning out sun, on which physical and chemical forces of nature have been reduced to such a degree that has allowed for the emergence of organic matter and therefore for life. Nevertheless, our star has not yet come to rest. It bubbles and hisses under the surface; the great tectonic plates move, leading to volcanic eruptions and earthquakes. Added to that are excessive heat, cold, and wind, which cause an increasing number of natural catastrophes for all living beings on earth. These natural disasters can also be traumatising for people, and in fact add to the burden in traumatised and traumatising societies, increasing the amount of traumatised people. Forest fires, floods and earthquakes, are natural phenomena not caused by people. However, it cannot be disputed that humankind overall destroys nature due to rapid population growth, striving for profits, and an addiction to consumption as a trauma diversion strategy. Too many trees are being chopped down and too much carbon dioxide is being produced and blown into the atmosphere. Humankind, therefore, is creating the climate change that is leading to fiercer storms and greater floods. This is another consequence of trauma-survival strategies, which only look for short-term solutions and relief, and thereby are destroying many sensitive eco systems.

We humans have enough to do coping with natural disasters, to keep recovering from them and not allow them to discourage us. Do we really need the additional destruction of our cities and living spaces through military and economic wars that also make our inner, psychological landscapes increasingly uninhabitable?

Constructiveness or destructiveness?

Initially for us humans our world is a universe of interpersonal relationships. We do have the opportunity to live in constructive or destructive relationships, and in light of the fundamental conflicts of human existence briefly outlined above, we can make the decision to treat each other in a friendly or a violent way with regards to our personal, economical, or political connections, in respect of ...

- conflicts of interests between parents and children,
- different sexual urges and needs for love in couple relationships,
- desires to want what others have,
- the tendency to react with anger and violence when we feel frightened or threatened.

It is therefore possible ...

- to show children love and kindness instead of rejection and indifference,
- to practice a cooperative relationship instead one of dominance and submission,
- to strive for economic collaboration instead of engaging in competition, monopolisation, and exploitation,
- to assume global responsibility, to respect the international law, and to promote peaceful coexistence instead of counting on rivalry, violence, and war to gain short-term, ephemeral national advantages.

In constructive relationships the 'We' is the sum of 'I' plus 'You': We = I + You. Then, 'We' has a different quality than 'I' and 'You' alone can have. A family is constructive if mother, father, and children can each live out their own needs, interests, and peculiarities.

In destructive relationships, the 'We' is the result of dominance and submission. This 'We' is then only qualitatively more than the 'I' and the 'You' alone; it is also abstract and has no content: We = I = You. A concept such as the 'European Union' is not constructive as long as it is only interested in uniting as many countries as possible in one common single market in which the economically stronger nations dominate the financially weaker ones. Or, if the whole EU project is intended to be a competing power bloc against the USA and China.

There cannot be national solutions to the problems of the whole of humankind. If we were to strive for constructiveness, the economical and political world order and the dealing with nature would look completely different, than when destruction and competition are the driving forces behind all our actions. With a constructive attitude, we try to create win-win situations. A destructive attitude leads to win-lose or lose-lose situations. With a destructive and competitive stance, the psychological as well as material resources are largely applied to the destruction of other people, turning them into victims. In this way, we can see that traumatising perpetrator-victim relationships on all four levels of dependency develop repeatedly, with their particular short and long-term consequences. In this scenario there will be no end to this destructiveness. On the contrary, the spiral of violence will continue to escalate.

Today, constructivity as a principle for interpersonal forms of relationship is still more of a wishful idea than a common reality. It is grim to realise that humans continuously and systematically traumatise each other at all possible levels of relationship.

Thus we continuously create new trauma victims and new trauma perpetrators ...

- on a political level,
- in the domain of economics,

- in our partnerships,
- in our families.

It is easy to see from the biographical details of tyrants, terrorists, economic oligarchs, and political dictators that children, who became victims of their parents perpetration, will go on to cause great damage in their adult partnerships, economic life, and politics by becoming perpetrators themselves (Miller, 2006; Gruen, 2015 a, b). We ruthlessly repeat in later relationships attachment patterns established with violent or abusive parents. Childhood trauma victims turn into adult trauma perpetrators who apply their early infantile trauma survival mechanisms recklessly as adults to themselves and others.

That is a fact that has shown itself to be valid during the numerous psychotherapies that I have conducted with my clients. I can clearly confirm this in my own biography too. Competitive orientation and aggression are not 'natural' or 'normal' human characteristics. They are the consequences of trauma. They are caused by 'competitive systems' created by society, implemented through power hierarchies, and forcefully sustained. In ancient times, this was the condition of the state of Sparta in a particularly cruel way. The Spartans' complete social organisation was aimed at the cultivation of warriors. National Socialism in Germany had the same aim with its educational motto that children should be "tough as leather, hard as Krupp's steel, and swift as greyhounds".

To fight or adapt?

A child either builds a safe and trusting bond with his mother and father which he can convert into self-confidence, bringing this into all his other relationships, or he can develop a 'combat mode', or an 'avoidance mode' in relationship with his traumatised parents. The combative mode teaches the child that in order to receive attention from his mentally and emotionally dissociated parents he has to get angry and make a noise. The avoidance mode teaches the child that he has to hold back on his emotional expressions in order to avoid causing his traumatised parents to dissociate further and not provoke their aggression. Therefore he becomes outwardly well-behaved, quiet, and 'adjusted', but internally he is highly stressed, hopeless, and full of anger and negativity.

The relational bond of the child to his mother or father can have a different quality; if the child is fortunate, he can develop a loving and supportive relationship bond with at least one parent. However, since traumatised people are often mutually attracted to each other, many children have no option but to choose between the fight and avoidance mode. Since the bond with the mother is the earlier, and therefore a deeper psychologically formative bond, this early-developed pattern is repeated in other relationships.

When children have experienced the connection to their parents as a relationship of power, control, and submission, a basic mistrust of other people is difficult to overcome. Therefore, people who changed their roles from childhood trauma victim to adult trauma perpetrator occupy all social, economical, and political institutions in society. In this way, a negative social spiral perpetually increases.

According to the psychological resonance principle, people with trauma-survival skills attract others with similar trauma-survival skills, and people more in their healthy space conversely will keep their distance from those who act through trauma-survival strategies.

With the example of Adolf Hitler, we can see clearly how this severely traumatised human pulled millions of people into the abyss of his psychotrauma through his trauma-survival strategies. Many generations have subsequently suffered the consequences of the wars he masterminded. However, Hitler was only able to implement the lunacy of his trauma-survival strategies because most of his followers were as traumatised as he was. Thus, they easily allowed themselves to be manipulated into his perpetrator-victim dynamic. Someone with a healthy psyche would neither think of, nor do the abhorrent actions that the National Socialists did. Someone with a healthy psyche, on the other hand would not allow himself or herself to be deceived, or dragged into such utterly senseless and hopeless fights. Propaganda is only fruitful when it falls onto the fertile ground of a traumatised psyche.

So I think that it is not status or class that causes splits at a social or global level. An employer is not a perpetrator per se, and an employee is not a victim per se. A politician is not necessarily by nature a power-obsessed tyrant. Men are not perpetrators of violence per se, and women are not always affectionate by nature. Psychotraumas turn people into victims to start with, and then confuse their psyche to the point that they become perpetrators whilst refusing to acknowledge it.

These traumatisations deeply split people within themselves, and then result in irreconcilable divisions in communities. This much should be clear to us by now: the human psyche does not change for the better through aggression and the withdrawal of love. It will only be even further traumatised.

Existence and consciousness

If we as humans want to have better relationships with each other, we first have to change our relationship with ourselves. It is utterly pointless to demand changes in attitudes, thought and behaviour in others if we are not willing to change and develop ourselves.

The sciences that are concerned with external relationships, the natural sciences, political science, sociology, economics, and business management, generally do not have a good understanding of the human psyche. The sciences that concern themselves with people and their behaviour, i.e. psychology and education, often disregard political and economic circumstances in their thinking. However, the influence of the individual on society and vice versa have to work hand in hand, so that we do not continue to lead each other down the familiar road to ruin. If we change our behaviour, circumstances will change. If circumstances change, our behaviour will also change. This holds true for better and for worse. Structural changes alone (new laws, new institutions, new buildings, roads, new technologies ...) achieve nothing positive in a society that does not at the same time address the feelings and thinking of people for the better. Whereas an evolution and increase in awareness leads to new societal structures, because people are no longer willing to live in old and bad circumstances. Our consciousness and resulting theories determine the way we live. False theories and perspectives lead to false and destructive forms of existence.

4
Traumatic personal experiences

The damage that a person suffers can be more or less significant; we recover from smaller incidents of harm, for example, the theft of our mobile phone, after a short while. However, there are also damages that stay with us permanently. That is clearly observable with the physical consequences of violence; the limb shot off during a war will not grow back. With psychological damage this is less observable. What is needed then is a proper examination of the phenomenon of 'psychotrauma' in order to understand why early childhood neglect or sexual traumatisation can lead with certainty to lifelong psychological damage. These wounds do not heal over time, but instead escalate throughout life even though, and especially when, the person actually thinks he is fine.

The harm becomes a traumatising event if the person experiences himself as helpless and powerless through another person's act or failure to act. If, in addition, all his or her automatically activated stress reactions – 'fight or flight' – do not help, but instead make the situation worse, then emergency responses such as becoming motionless, freezing, dissociation, and splitting of the personality become necessary in order to increase the possibility of survival. For instance, if a child cries when he is hit, and his crying makes the perpetrator even more aggressive, this child has to suppress his feelings as much as possible to avoid more beating.

Since the psyche, as already mentioned above, principally serves two main purposes, the preservation of the self and the preservation of the species, traumas can potentially occur derived from these. There are on the one hand traumas that concern physical self-preservation (for example if I suffer a car accident or if I am assaulted by someone). These are accompanied by mortal fear that my life is in danger. On the other hand there are traumas that concern the preservation of the species (for example if a mother loses her child), causing the unbearable pain of loss.

Body-psyche split

Traumatic experiences can force people into a body-psyche split, which seems to concur with the dualistic idea that mind and body are separate from each other. The psyche has to abandon the body to its fate and save itself by retreating into a world of ideas disconnected from the body: I think, therefore I am!

Through trauma experiences we find ourselves in a state of a split psyche, in which perception, feeling, thinking, wanting, remembering, and acting no longer work as one unit, but exist independently from each other in the processing of information about the real world. The self-organisation of the psychic system ceases to function properly.

This split between psyche and body, and between the various psychic functions, can no longer resolve itself, especially if the person still has to live in the traumatising situation, for example in a violent family situation, an exploitative business, or a political dictatorship.

My own first hand experience as a child of cleanliness training, to use the potty instead of nappies, has put my bladder under permanent stress. In an exploration of this topic I became aware of how as a two-year-old child I suffered many beatings for having wet my bed, resulting in my psyche splitting in the face of the threat of violence if it happened again, and the unloving treatment I experienced when having my nappy changed. One part of me felt helpless and totally exposed, while another part tried to calm myself through rocking back and forth, and a further part wanted to stay as much as possible awake so that I would not wet my bed again. In this process, my experience was that it took such a mental effort that I became totally hot in my head. I had had to surrender to a situation that I was at that age unable to consciously control.

While in the state of trauma, the human psyche comes into a fundamental contradiction with its function. Instead of giving a person clear access to reality as it is, the psyche now has to make sure that the person does not recognise fully the reality in which they are at that moment.

This has huge consequences for the entire life of the traumatised person; they lose contact with the outer reality as well as their inner world. From that moment on they have to cope with an enormous reduction of their reference to reality. They have to invent substitute worlds and realities in their head ('head-births'), to try to compensate for the lack of access to actual reality. These fantasy worlds have the advantage that the person appears, at least to him or herself, to have control over their life circumstances, and they can see these illusionary worlds as more tolerable than the real world.

For example, a prostitute may imagine that she is offering her body for sex out of choice, and that she would thereby have control over her client, something that was not the case in her childhood, when her father sexually traumatised her daily. It is likely that all prostitutes were sexually abused as children. Nevertheless, this illusion of control does not lead to her having a good life. She is now constantly being sexually traumatised by her own actions and with her own approval every day, physically as well as psychologically. Then she has to listen to the collective cynicism that after all, now she is doing it out of free choice.

Psychotraumas cause the trauma conditions to be permanently stored in the psyche and the body. The unbearable reality has to be located deep within his self and there it continues to exist, even if the outer reality is over. Therefore, traumatised people are in a permanent state of stress, having to expend an enormous amount of energy in the suppression of their trauma experiences, which continually surface from the body into consciousness. Traumatised people have to make a tremendous effort all the time to prevent the intrusion of traumatic memories into their conscious perception. It is the only way in which they can reasonably cope with their everyday life.

Constant stress and panic prevent any further development

of their healthy 'I', making access to their healthy 'I' completely impossible at times. Traumatised people continue to be completely overwhelmed and controlled by their perceptions and feelings, being largely guided by what they perceive in their outer world, and by whatever can distract them from what is actually happening in their body. In these situations it is very easy for traumatised people to make decisions and do things that can cause further damage to themselves and to others. They find it difficult to think and plan, and in this condition they cannot take responsibility for their actions. They re-stage their trauma violations repeatedly.

In summary, this means that a traumatised psyche finds it difficult to distinguish clearly and reliably inside from outside, then from now, I from you, and reality from fiction. Traumatised people start to be stressed and agitated on the slightest provocation; at the same time they often find themselves in immensely dangerous situations without having the perception to grasp the seriousness of the situation. Trauma means that we use yesterday's patterns of survival in order to overcome today's problems. The current external society is experienced with reference to the internal experiences from the past. Previous inner fears from the past are projected onto the outer reality of the now. The past continues to live on relentlessly in the here and now. The distinction between the self and other people fails; the unfamiliar is experienced as one's own, and what belongs to oneself is experienced as unfamiliar. I feel like you, and you think you are I. Moreover, you believe that you can make decisions about me even though you have no control over yourself!

Trauma Triad

In my experience, many people do not simply suffer individual psychotraumas; their entire life destiny is formed by a triple negative omen: they are not wanted, not loved, and not protected. That is the fatal trauma-triad, with which many people have to cope from early childhood. In particular, it is the unborn children, the newly born, and post birth babies that are the most vulnerable, and the least able to defend themselves against the trauma of being the victim of rejection, lovelessness and violence. Due to the absolute dependence of the child on their mother, these newly created humans are easily distressed if they are not wanted, not loved, and not protected (Figure 2).

The Trauma Triad

Not wanted!
Not loved!
Not protected!

Figure 2: The Trauma Triad

Trauma induced splitting of the psyche

The self-regulatory function of the psychic system as a whole can no longer work after traumatic experiences, therefore, each trauma leads to a splitting of the psyche into three different parts (Figure 3):

- The healthy part, in which the psyche continues to grasp reality and is able to manage and regulate itself.
- The traumatised parts in which unbearable feelings caused by the trauma situation – fear, pain, anger, shame, and disgust – are encapsulated.

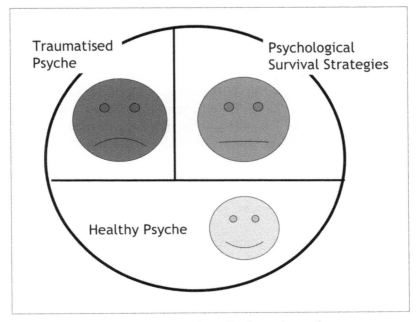

Figure 3: The human psyche split through psychotrauma

- The trauma-survival strategies, by which the unbearable reality of the trauma disappears into a fog, is hidden, ignored, no longer felt, thought of or remembered, and instead is replaced with an illusionary world.

The loss of ones ability to self-regulate goes hand in hand with the loss of reference to reality; blind actions accompanied by incessant talk take the place of considered action.

Since these trauma-survival strategies are lifesaving in an acute situation they have a great influence on the later life of the traumatised person. Even if there is no threat, these psychological structures insist on behaving as if the mortal danger still existed. The affected person's quality of life then suffers enormously, because instead of freely perceiving and feeling, he constantly has to do and act. The traumatised person lives in a chronic mood of over excitation. If the trauma-survival strategies were lifesaving at the time of the traumatising experience, later on they can literally cost him his life, especially since the suppression of feelings has to be maintained, and even some normal healthy impulses are perceived as dangerous and need to be fought and suppressed. Therefore, stress is omnipresent in traumatised societies, in partnerships, families, schools, in companies, and in politics. Equally manifold are the attempts to deal with the stress, for example by smoking, drinking, eating, consuming medication, yoga exercises, relaxation techniques, massages, hypnosis. These may reduce stress in the short term, but in the long term they may even increase the stress. Fitness exercises and sport, calorie conscious eating or the controlled use of addictive substances can in themselves become a source of stress.

On the other hand, there can be the experience of bleakness and boredom because of the emotional numbing caused by trauma, and the resulting inner emptiness. This in turn encourages addictive behaviour such as consumerism, search for distractions, or the merging with one's mobile phone and the constant waiting for fresh news, emails or 'likes'. This leads to the paradoxical situation of trying to overcome the older stresses in the body by creating new stresses.

Something similar holds true for the medical perspective, which raises the stress levels even further using medicines and operations. Thus, children who are diagnosed with 'hyperactivity' or 'ADHD' are put into a temporary physiological state of exhaustion with stimulating substances ('amphetamines'), which will last for a while until the inner stress conditions once again return with the decrease of the drug's effect. Then the child needs the next pill until eventually the brain structure is permanently damaged, and this may threaten early Parkinsons symptoms (Hüther and Bonney, 2002).

Indeed, these children suffer from an 'attention deficit disorder' in the sense that they do not receive the attention and care from their traumatised parents which they needed as infants, babies, and in early childhood. Therefore, they split off their fears, anger and pain at a very early age and come to focus only on the external world. Once this splitting off from the original feelings has taken place even 1,000 'likes' on their Facebook or Twitter accounts later on do not help to compensate for this deficit of attention and reassurance. It is a bottomless pit and nowadays quickly leads to an addiction to the Internet. Two hours without an Internet connection and children and young people become nervous, irritable, and aggressive.

Surviving instead of living

The trauma emergency mechanism has to banish unbearable feelings and the truth from consciousness. Thoughts that are devoid of feelings lose their touch with reality. Such thoughts become more and more abstract. They stand above reality and view life from a meta-position. In its mildest form, this can become what appears to be a scientific intellectualism with the highest accuracy requirements. In an extreme case, it can lead to incessant circling of thinking, to the wildest random connections of ideas, and a constant waterfall of words, which in psychiatric nomenclature is described as 'schizophrenia'. Dissociated talking is difficult to endure, as are the practical actions that follow it.

The Psychotrauma Biography

The earlier a person becomes a victim of trauma the more lasting are the consequences for his life. It is all the more likely that his entire life represents a progressive trauma biography. Because of his traumatising childhood experiences he later emerges as a trauma perpetrator in his partnerships, his parenthood, in his connection with the economy, and politics. Those who are unable to exit their trauma biography will not find inner peace. The older they get the worse their mental state becomes and the clearer physical symptoms will present themselves.

The trauma biography begins with the 'trauma of identity', continues with the 'trauma of love', and often with the 'trauma of sexuality'. This leads almost inevitably to the 'trauma of

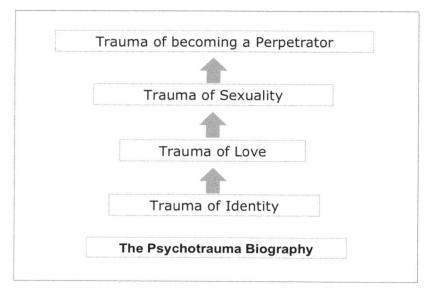

Figure 4: The psychotrauma biography in its four
developmental stages

becoming a perpetrator oneself' (see figure 4). This sequence of
traumas follows the developmental logic of the human psyche.
The four different types of psychotraumas I will briefly explain
as follows:

The trauma of identity

Someone who lives, even though his creators (his parents)
wanted that he should not exist, comes into a fundamental
conflict. He has to confirm his existence to his own parents. He
has to assert his life against the '*No*' of his mother and/or father.
How does a child manage that? How does he succeed in staying
alive, with massive feelings of rejection while in his mother's
womb, and perhaps even after attempted abortions?

According to my observations during therapeutic processes
with clients, we can only survive these conditions if we surrender
the emotional connection with our self, with our own wishes, our

own needs, and with our own body. An early split takes place in which mortal fears and the pain of rejection are compartmentalised, and our healthy 'I' goes into a dormant state. Our healthy will to live grows weary very early on and we replace it by a stubborn will to survive. This will to survive forces us into making ourselves as inconspicuous as possible, expressing minimal vigour, and acting in a way that the mother may not even notice that the growing child inside her is there. The unborn child already learns how to adapt to the mother so that she notices him as little as possible. Even his heartbeat he perceives as threatening since that draws attention to him. For the child his survival depends on being as unobtrusive as possible in utero, hiding within the womb, and taking on the mother's psyche as a cloak of invisibility during his unavoidable development: I (child) am you (mum)!

This self-abandonment and process of self-adjustment to fit with the mother has to be continued after birth in order to give the mother as little opportunity as possible to reject the child. The child develops a disguised identity based on his mother's rejection, her attributions and criticisms. Surviving in this way the unwanted and unloved child seeks salvation by attuning to his mother, and so to his trauma perpetrator. He has no choice. The relationship formula 'We = I + my mother' is changed to 'We = I = my mother. This results in the paradox that the constructive self is perceived as alien, and the destructive alien (the mother) is perceived as myself. Even my 'I' has to be fought actively against in order to identify with my mother .

Every child carries an essential '*yes*' to life and to his own existence after the unifying of ovum and sperm. If the child then feels his mother's rejection, his vital energy is consumed in finding some connection around the 'No' of the mother, to the point that it becomes unclear to the child who is who? Who says 'yes' and who says 'no'? The 'No' of the mother becomes the reference point of the child's life. Even in his adult life, the child finds it extremely difficult to outgrow this (Figure 5).

This primary trauma, in which the child's will to live is confronted by a principle 'No' from the outside, can develop into different forms of self-attacking, for example so-called auto-immune diseases or 'cancer'. Also often present in an unwanted person is the suicidal thought that it would be best if I were not here. This suicidal ideation can intensify if further traumas are added to the person's biography. Therefore, if a further trauma occurs and the person's trauma-survival strategies fail to manage it, there is an increased risk of actual suicide. Suicidal tendencies can also be expressed through life threatening and self-harming actions, or with persistent drug abuse.

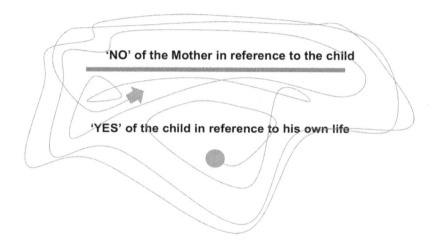

Figure 5: The rejected child, with his/her original 'Yes' to life, forced to take on the mother's 'No' in reference to her child

Like all early processes, these occurrences happen unconsciously, and that is why people who suffer from a trauma of identity search in all later relationships, in addition to their ongoing relationship with their mother, for what they had to give up: vital energy, zest for life, even the will to live. They often have the feeling that alone they are not viable, that they cannot survive on their own. Any relationship with another person becomes for them a substitute 'I', a compulsive imperative for their survival, and that also means that there must always be a relationship. Being alone and not in a relationship is perceived as life threatening and pointless.

It is for this reason that there is a great need to identify with anybody or anything: I am a wife, a German, a Christian, a Jew, a Moslem, a football club supporter and so on. This translates into external things having a higher purpose than oneself, like marriage, the family, the nation, God, the football club, the job. People will sacrifice their lifetime, their money, their energy, in an effort to turn the external into an apparent identity, and by doing this they make themselves invisible and unimportant, hiding behind masks and roles. In the most extreme cases some people will even sacrifice their life for such an external identification.

I have a painful first hand experience of trying to cover up my trauma of identity by supporting a football club. In my childhood, my mother's youngest brother was a strong role model for me. He was a tank and truck driver during his military service. He already had his own car, which was still a great rarity in the countryside in Germany at that time. And he was a fan of the Nürnberg Football Club. When I was eight years old he often took me and some friends to the Nürnberg stadium by car. Those were big journeys and adventures for a small boy from the countryside. My devotion to my uncle in itself made me a 'club' fan, especially when the 'Club' won the ninth German football championship in 1968. I idolized the 'Club' and collected everything I could find about this club in the newspapers. To get the autograph of a famous player filled me with greatest joy. To have this small share of the glamour of stardom was like being on cloud nine for this little country lad. Every Saturday I listened to the radio broadcasts 'Today at the stadium'. If the 'Club' won, the weekend and the following week were safe for me. 'My Club' provided me with happiness, and I was accepted amongst my friends. However, if the 'Club' lost the match of the week it was a personal disgrace for me. I felt an incredible sense of shame.

Unfortunately, in that respect there was significantly more reason for shame than for pride in the years after 1968. The 'Club'

71

went down from the premier league to the regional league nine times. Instead of dreaming of the championship again, it meant shaking in my boots until the last day of the games in the Bundesliga, hoping that the 'Club' would not sink further. Sometimes it would give me heart palpitations and an attack of the nerves as though my own life depended on it. Today I know that the defeats and descents of this 'Club' triggered my own trauma of identity over and over again.

Even in later years, when my critical thinking made it clear that this unshakable loyalty to my football club was crazy, the little boy inside me could not stop, because he needed the identification in order to ignore his own needs and not have to give up the yearning of his infantile love. I was ashamed of my attachment, which I had carried over from my childhood days into my adult life. I tried to suppress the constant impulse to pay attention to the scores of the 'Club', but kept relapsing. I also tried to hide my football addiction from my girlfriends and from my wife. I only later realised how the trauma of identity can lead to living a double life. The seemingly adult façade, which I lived externally, had to share its psyche with the small boy whose personal happiness and sadness were dependent on the wins and losses of his club. This little Franz inside me was dependent on the behaviours and accomplishments of those football players, without them suspecting how much he loved and needed them. In this way, my trauma of identity developed into a trauma of love. I outsourced and expanded the symbiotic involvement with my mother and my father onto a football club.

I was able to give up this identification through therapeutic work on my trauma of identity. It became crystal clear to me, when reading Alfie Kohn's book about competition (Kohn, 1989), how sport in particular serves to make competition and blind partiality socially normal. Already at birth the backpack of national and religious belonging is strapped to the small traumatised child, and so one thinks of oneself as being more special and better than others who belong to a different nation or religion. During my lifetime, I have put further stones into my backpack 'voluntarily', by sharing the excitement of competition with 'my' athlete friends and teams, just to have a sense of belonging. It is a big relief for me

to take this competition backpack off and to make cooperation
more preferable than competition.

For someone who has suffered a trauma of identity nothing
is obvious. Breathing, heartbeat, body temperature, body
sensation, eating, excreting, being able to move, having their
own needs ... everything is questioned because this person is
constantly questioning himself, and believes he can only exist if
he puts himself in the shoes of others and puts their needs before
his.

Is the incidence of a trauma of identity because of the
parents' rejection of the child an exceptional situation? I am
afraid not. There are many reasons why children are unwanted.
This is shown by the high abortion rates of about 50 million
worldwide per year. Women are often forced to have sex, and
many women get pregnant at an unsuitable time in their life: they
are still at school or university, they are not making enough
money, or they are not in a steady relationship. Pregnancy
before marriage in the past was generally seen as a disgrace, and
still is for women in many countries. Or a woman becomes
pregnant even though she does not want to bring another child
into the world and have to raise it; perhaps she already has
several children. In addition, it is understandable that a woman
does not want a child that is the consequence of rape.

It can also be that the gender of the child does not suit the
parents, because there is already a boy, so the second child
should be a girl. When there was a single child policy in China,
most parents wanted a boy rather than a girl. In India, too,
parents usually want male offspring because later they will
receive a dowry for him, whilst a high price has to be paid for the
marriage of a daughter.

With traumatised parents the wish to have children is often a
trauma survival strategy, to fill up their inner emptiness and
loneliness, perhaps motivated by their wish to conform to social
standards and expectations: wanting to be better parents than
their own parents, wanting to compensate for their own lack of
identity by taking on the identity of a mother or father. In all of
these cases, it is not about the particular child. Right from the

start the child has to fulfil the function of being a trauma survival aid for her mother and/or father. That can lead to absurd situations. One of my students described the case study of a 40-year old woman who still wanted to fulfil her wish to have children. After many attempts, artificial insemination was finally successful. She had a twin pregnancy but one child died before birth. The mother then placed the surviving child into a full-time nursery when it was only 10 months old. Why then did she want a child, when she gave him away so early?

If a mother is ambivalent as to whether she wants a child or not, the child has to exist with a sword of Damocles over his head; the fear that the mother might turn her thumb down is permanently present. I notice with many clients that they would rather cling to the idea that their mother had partially wanted them, than to admit the truth of not being wanted. This way it becomes impossible for them to recognise the perpetration against themselves by their mother and she remains under their skin, like an irritant they cannot get rid of. Unfortunately the attitude that 'your mother certainly loved you, even if she was unable to show it, owing to her own problems', is encouraged by a trauma-blind society and by some psychotherapists. So the responsibility is placed on the child to discover the 'hidden maternal love' rather than come to terms with the truth. Many years of frustrating therapy can be spent on this issue.

The trauma of love

Every child loves his or her mother, and relates to her entirely through his emotions. Since he is existentially dependent on his mother, every child tries to give his mother love, and hopes to receive love back. That is a primary infantile instinct, which no child can consciously stop. However, because of their own traumatisations, many mothers are not able to accept this infantile love; they feel threatened by the needs and emotional expressions of their child, and are scared that they will end up with even deeper trauma feelings. Therefore, the mother will try everything to suppress the child's emotional expressions by ignoring, by rocking the child, through feeding, appeasement, strict or sad glances, or with direct violence.

These maternal reactions are so frightening and painful for the child that he makes every effort to suppress the expression of his feelings as best he can. Consequently, very early on children try to figure out how they are supposed to be so that their mother is not angry with them. Since the child cannot know that the mother is emotionally rejecting because of her own traumatisation, the child believes that it is his fault that his mother does not love him. The child feels that gaining his mother's love hinges on his ability to control his feelings, to understand his mother better and meet her needs, and relieve her from her troubles and distress. Thus children unconsciously, and as they grow up, increasingly, assume responsibility for their mothers' traumas, which forces them to take on the role of mothering their own mother. Something similar can repeat itself in relation to the child's father.

Children, who are forced into a trauma of love, because of their own trauma of identity, remain caught in this trap. The less they feel loved, the more effort they have to make. They will idolise their mother, and can never really get away from her. All their lives they remain in the role of a child in relation to their mother, and focused on the objective that one day their mother will be redeemed from her suffering, and will then accept and return the love of the child. This inner programme can continue even after the mother has died.

The life energy of a child that is neither wanted nor loved is consumed largely in working through the trauma-survival strategies of her parents, and especially of her mother. For the child it is like being snared with her own infantile love in the barbed wire of the maternal or paternal trauma survival strategies. It is alarming to witness the power traumatised mothers have over their children to the extent that the child dares not express her own feelings.

For me, as a ten year old, my feelings and needs finally came to a frozen state, when my mother threatened to commit suicide; to demonstrate this she hung a rope on a beam in the attic and placed a chair underneath. Every time she went up there I was scared stiff, and then relieved when she came back down.

People who are stuck in a trauma of love continue to search for the ideal mother, one that finally makes them feel wanted and loved, throughout their life. Friendships and partnerships suffer from the pressure of such high expectations, which are doomed to fail, since in these scenarios, too, the process of emotional repression is restaged and repeated. Someone else will never be able to replace this missing love. Moreover, in every intimate relationship the person is hindered by his infantile survival strategies of suppressing his own feelings. If it is not possible for someone to win back the abandoned 'I', to develop his own will, and to accept and love himself wholeheartedly, then he will not be able to love anyone else in a healthy way. Even in long-standing partnerships, he cannot shake off the basic feeling that he is lonely and abandoned. For him the world of love chiefly consists of illusions of love and the sorrows of love.

Workaholism is a trauma survival strategy that goes well with the trauma of love. I made myself useful to others through my work performance. I did not work for myself but rather for others. I sacrificed myself with great commitment in order to appeal to others, to impress them, to help them, and to save them whilst not paying attention to my own needs and without showing my true feelings.

The trauma of sexuality

If I am in the state of 'trauma of love', there is a great danger that my sexuality, too, is deployed in my futile search for love and security, and that this will allow me to be abused by others. With my sexuality, I try to get something that sexuality cannot provide. That is how many people slide from the 'trauma of love' into the next trauma: the 'trauma of sexuality'. This kind of trauma is not an exception, but is spread like an epidemic worldwide. The international '#metoo' movement on social networks makes this clearly visible. Since the 'trauma of identity' is so frequent, the 'trauma of love' and the 'trauma of sexuality' are also the rule rather than the exception.

Because children who were not loved or protected by their parents are in need of bodily contact and touch, they become easy prey for sexual perpetrators in their environment. The perpetrators, out of their own lack of love and in their own frustrated infantile needs for physical closeness, feel attracted to vulnerable children. They will offer a child the body contact for which he or she yearns. The child takes the *'yes'* of the perpetrator at face value and includes this seeming saviour into its psychological structure. The child feels noticed and, at least initially, enjoys the physical contact and touch. In this way, he identifies with and enmeshes himself with the perpetrator, who by his tricks obtains the goodwill of the emotionally starved child. The perpetrator, because of his superior mental and body strength, can satisfy his sexual arousal with the child repeatedly.

When a father sexually traumatises his own child, he does so on the basis of his 'identity' and 'love traumas'. He is fixated on the child and uses the sexual contact as one of his trauma-survival strategies. Perpetrators, who are sexually invasive, due to their own trauma biography, have no feelings for their own body, or awareness of its limitations. They cannot feel where their body begins and where it ends, and so they are apt to monopolise someone else's body in order to feel themselves. On the other side, the child already feels completely separated from her healthy 'I', and feels dependent on any physical contact with her parents. Since, as a rule, the mothers of sexually traumatised children are emotionally unavailable and physically rejecting, the father is the only remaining person with whom some physical contact may be possible. The child desires her father despite his sexual violence. While one part of the child clings needily onto him, another part is scared of him and would want to kill him because of his sexual actions. I have seen this dynamic in numerous therapy processes in groups as well as individual therapy sessions.

For all children it is utterly humiliating and shameful to be treated as a sexual object. Additionally, the sexual acts that a sexual perpetrator carries out on a child are often extremely painful and disgusting. So, the sexually traumatised child has to split off her physical pain, her shame, disgust, her voice, and feelings of anger towards the perpetrator. The disbelief that their own father or grandfather, or even their mother, could do these things serves the child as a survival strategy. Instead, the idea is held on to that it would be impossible for the perpetrator to assume such an immense guilt. After all, he had also been kind and supportive.

Because the familiar and societal environment systematically ignores the sexual traumatisation of children, many suffer a continuing ordeal. I have worked with a number of women who were sexually traumatised orally as children. When, because of that, their tonsils became inflamed and swollen, they were without further ado taken to hospitals where their tonsils were cut out, sometimes without anaesthesia. Consequently, they had to carry with them the additional fears of death and abandonment throughout their entire life, and were robbed of important components of their immune system.

Unfortunately many people who use the term 'sexual abuse' for the sexual traumatisation of children have little knowledge of the psychological dynamics involved, and the profound and lasting damage such experiences can cause in the human psyche. The effects of sexual trauma continue to affect the psyche until the trauma can be fully recognised by the person concerned, and by her therapist.

In many families, women have been victims of sexual violence for many generations. Then, as sexually traumatised mothers, they can neither protect their daughters from sexual perpetrators, nor are they emotionally and physically available for their sons. Their sons, who already during the pregnancy to some extent are perceived by their mother as a perpetrator, are likely then to grow up as the next generation of sex offenders. I work in many countries, and in none of them have I had the impression that they have the epidemic of childhood sexual traumatisation under control, not legally, medically, psychotherapeutically or socio-pedagogically.

Sexually traumatised women are also more likely to be sexually invasive towards their children and grandchildren. They unconsciously restage their own infantile experiences with children. Their own confused sexual boundaries mean that they are unable to distinguish between love and sexuality in contact with their daughters and sons.

The issue of sexual violence then continues in adult relationships. Sex is frequently demanded or enforced. Partners and spouses are seen as property whose sexual use is an entitlement.

Circumcision is another traumatising action performed on millions of boys and girls. Many women experience violence during their pregnancy and delivery, and thus are further sexually traumatised (Mundlos, 2015).

The 'trauma of sexuality' pervades our society in the forms of prostitution, pornography, and sexual harassment within and outside of the work place. Mass rape during war and as part of military occupation represents the extremes of sexual traumatisation. Traumatised soldiers are left with no inhibitions, acting out their sexual urges on defenceless women and children of the politically defined 'enemy'.

The trauma of becoming a perpetrator

The trauma of becoming a perpetrator oneself is very likely included in everyone's trauma biography. The trauma triad, of being unwanted, unloved, and unprotected, produces trauma victims with survival strategies that in one way or another turn a trauma victim into a trauma perpetrator.

Because we repress our own victimhood, denying and refusing to acknowledge that we have been a trauma victim, we restage this every day by making other people victims of our actions. For example, even small children may act out the sexual assault that they have experienced themselves with other children; older or physically stronger siblings terrorise their younger and weaker brothers and sisters. This gives them some short-term relief from their own experience of powerlessness into a position of superiority and power. When the unbearable trauma feelings of helplessness and terror rise up within them, they numb themselves in order not to feel, and they lash out blindly against others. The stronger the split-off pain, the stronger becomes the hatred and readiness to use violence against other people.

However, trauma perpetrators find it hard to bear the painful feelings of others, because that awakens their own split-off feelings, and so they have to banish those who express feelings from their perception, if necessary even kill them if they do not stop crying or screaming. However, even that does not really help them, since the trauma feelings inside them continue to exist and will be triggered again at the next opportunity. This then creates many new trauma victims, and the perpetrator continues to traumatise himself through his actions. The ultimate increase of this dynamic is that this can give rise to mass murders. It can become an obsession, and an addiction, to terrorise, humiliate, and stalk people. This is clear not just through understanding the history of German National Socialism, but it is easy to see that these tendencies exist worldwide. The cruel 'holy warriors' of ISIS fighting for an Islamic State are just one example.

The trauma biography, with its different types of traumas and comparative forms, perpetually develops increasing victim-perpetrator dynamics within the psyche of a person, which are inevitably transferred onto other people. The person is entangled with other people because of his traumas; he entangles others in his trauma biography. Once someone is captured by such perpetrator-victim dynamics, it is hard for them to be able to use their psyche for their own benefit. They will become increasingly controlled by destructive, instead of constructive, psychological strategies. Unfortunately, these strategies are constructed in such a way as to prevent their being deleted or stopped. Whilst traumatised people remain focused on the survival strategies of perpetration, they will fight tooth and nail against the realisation that they are traumatised themselves, that they are just as much a victim as they are a perpetrator. They strongly reject the idea of addressing their own psyche. As soon as someone points to their traumatisation they feel attacked and insulted. Like a computer that has been infected with a virus, such a person then relentlessly veers towards his psychological and physical maximum tolerance. This is the same as a threat that is known in the nuclear industry as maximum credible accident (MCA): if he does not come to his senses at some point, and find help to get out of the downward spiral of his trauma biography things will get even worse.

Existential trauma and the trauma of loss in the context of trauma biography

In my earlier publications (Ruppert, 2002; Ruppert, 2005) I asserted that existential trauma and the trauma of loss are fundamental trauma categories. Through the concept of the psychotrauma biography, it has now become clear to me that experiences of existential trauma and trauma of loss function differently depending on which phase of his trauma biography a person is in.

- Thus, a traumabiography can begin with an attempted abortion, which, if it fails, is an existential trauma experience for the developing child. When, as an adult, the person has a serious car accident, it can be a trauma per se, but it can also leave the person severely shaken because this current trauma event triggers the original trauma, the survival of the attempted abortion.
- If someone has become a trauma perpetrator, they may potentially be so numbed in their survival strategies that even a present day extreme existential trauma experience no longer shakes them. This situation, for example, is restaged in action films all the time.
- Traumas of loss function differently, too, depending on how many trauma survival strategies a person has already established within himself. If a child loses his mother, to whom he was able to form a loving relationship prenatally, the impact on his psyche will be different to that of the child who has already sensed in the mother's womb that he was not wanted.

- A person who predominantly lives in a 'trauma of love' is less able to mourn and recover from the loss of those to whom she is close, because she has defined her identity primarily through her relationship with the person lost.
- Women who have had several abortions are likely to be traumatised by the first termination, and the experience of the loss of this aborted child. All the later abortions will be experienced in a state of strong dissociation.

Traumas as the cause of self-destructiveness

Ultimately, the traumatisation of our psyche forces us into all sorts of trauma survival strategies, making us do the most absurd things. Instead of making our life as comfortable as possible, ensuring a beautiful start in life for our children, creating a loving environment for them, using our skills and intelligence to produce beautiful and useful resources and freely expressing our creativity, we do exactly the opposite:

- Sexual intercourse, which could be beautiful and sensual for the parties involved, degenerates into the re-enactment of experiences as a victim, and with that into a perpetrator-victim power struggle, triggering pain, shame, and disgust.
- The process of birth, which requires a calm, gentle, and loving environment, is perverted into a bloody spectacle on the operating table.
- Many women actively seek violent men as partners, and keep returning to them even after excessive acts of violence, since that is what is familiar to them.
- Many men choose such women as partners on purpose, but they will not be loved by them, just as they were not loved by their mothers.
- Some people self-harm by cutting with razors; others destroy themselves with alcohol and/or drugs.
- Others still lose their mind, go insane, and finally kill themselves, since they cannot distance themselves from

their perpetrators, and are psychologically merged with them.

- As adults, we have a guilty conscience if we do not want to have contact with our mother or father, even though they may have made our life hell during our childhood, so we repeatedly allow ourselves to be violated by them.

- As workers, employees, and managers we accept an economic order that constantly puts us under pressure to perform, keeps our wages as low as possible, and continually threatens us with the loss of our job.

- We work and produce for an economy that puts more and more wealth into the hands of a few, the big players, and leaves the vast majority of people with instability and poverty. We put up with it because in our childhood we failed to gain a sense of self-worth.

- As citizens our fear of violence and chaos makes us voluntarily choose the very politicians who commission this chaos, curb our freedom, monitor and control our private world to the greatest degree possible, and even send us into war on spurious grounds and on the basis of obvious lies.

- On a political and economic level, we expend energy and effort destroying what we have built up earlier, because we have lost access to our own joy of life, and can only feel a kind of malicious joy if others have to suffer the same way that we have had to. How much time and effort for example does it take hackers to destroy and manipulate our computer programmes!

In all of these cases, people behave against their own, existential interests. They do not pay attention to their health, to eating well, to breathing clean air, to protecting themselves and their body from damage and violence, and to enjoying their life. Instead of wholeheartedly living and loving, they somehow survive, full of fear and suppressed rage, subordinated to other people and their alleged values, rules, and principles. Sometimes they even wait, hoping for a quick ending to their miserable and pointless life, and that someone else will do them the favour of killing them.

Therefore, we humans can be made into trauma victims and at the same time become trauma perpetrators. This mixture of being the perpetrator and being the victim produces a volatile, intra-psychic dynamic, which is often difficult to see through. Hence the following chapter will illuminate first the victim side and then the perpetrator side. Subsequently, I will discuss further how being a victim and perpetrator affect the psyche of the individual and the consequences this has for the societies in which these people live.

5
The perpetrator-victim dynamic

Psychotrauma-victims

By definition, a person becomes a trauma victim by sustaining damage that he cannot cope with due to insufficient physical and psychological resources. For one thing, the cause can be a natural phenomenon such as fire, hurricane, tsunami, or earthquake. Such events usually lead to a reaction of solidarity between the people affected and their environment, so that the consequence of a natural phenomenon is more likely to be limited to a physical and material aspects.

It is different when someone becomes a trauma victim through the actions of another person. Then, they cannot count on the solidarity of others who are loyal to the perpetrator. Such cases eventually lead to psychotrauma even if the body remains externally unharmed.

Generally, we can see that the greatest damage for a psychotrauma victim occurs when the perpetrator is a person on whom the victim is dependent. Even more: if the victim trusts the perpetrator and loves him, it becomes particularly bad. A small child that is rejected by his beloved mother and sexually traumatised by his beloved father suffers a super MCA (maximum credible accident). The splitting up of the victim's psyche becomes essential, and the victim has to give up his identity so that he can stay in relationship with the perpetrator, who continues to cause the child harm.

Even citizens of a nation state find themselves in a situation of relationship trauma. They have to witness how their government lies to them, and imposes lasting damage through terrorist activities staged by their secret services. If police and justice do not save people from becoming victims but actively protect the perpetrators, the whole society becomes increasingly crazy.

Human trauma victims are especially:

- children with permanent physical and psychological damage due to parental violence;
- partners with psychological wounds resulting from conflict between them;
- – people whose economic livelihoods are destroyed i.e. through expropriation of land and natural resources or through loss of earning potential as worker and employee,
- people whose living environments are continuously and systematically poisoned through the effects of state-owned and economic institutions,
- starving, injured, and sick people and their relatives, as a consequence of the use of state powers and of wars,
- police officers going into action during such conflicts and soldiers who are 'burned out' in wars.

The perpetrator of psychotrauma

An act that inflicts traumatising damage on another human being creates a trauma perpetrator. This can happen on a psychological level through lies, fraud, indignity, shame, degradation, and humiliation; on a material level, theft and robbery; on a physical level corporal violence, manslaughter or murder. Even someone who 'only' breaks into a house can inflict traumatising damage onto its owners. The living space is a person's safe place, and the loss of the sense of security can have serious, psychological long-term effects, even if the insurance compensates for the material damage.

Acts of omission such as the withholding of food, help, care, contact, or the protection from violence can also develop into trauma. For example, if parents do not give their children the physical contact, emotional closeness, and love that every child requires during the early developmental stages, they cause permanent psychological damage to the child, which can only be made up for by complex therapeutic measures later on in life.

A perpetrator can cause trauma directly, deliberately, and systematically. For example:

- Deliberately planned wars strategically create masses of trauma victims. This extreme form of traumatisation needs the prior programming of the victims, so that they become an obedient instrument for those interested in power and domination.
- With some economic projects, involving for example the exploitation of natural resources or the construction of nuclear power plants, the long lasting and irreversible destruction and contamination of the environment for humans and other living beings is consciously accepted despite the knowledge of the likely consequences. Someone who deliberately manipulates the emission values on cars, for example, directly becomes the perpetrator of those whose lungs are severely damaged by the resulting fine material particles.
- In partnerships, a man may marry a woman knowing that he can force her with physical violence to be available sexually whenever he wants her.
- Many children are emotionally and physically exploited by their parents by being 'wanted' children, but only to fullfill their parents needs.
- There are educators, teachers, and instructors in school, home, and other educational systems who enjoy being physically and emotionally abusive (Müller-Münch, 2012; Weiss, 2012).

In a way, I also experience being bombarded with unwanted e-mails as a perpetration. Moreover, even though digital spying is an expected process and thought of as 'normal', I would like to point out how invasive and perpetrator-like this is. It represents a severe breach of trust. Even though a person may not be directly traumatised by it, the clearing of a person's bank account of money, or coming under the scrutiny of intelligence services, or having his professional existence destroyed by a social smear campaign can be traumatic and are forms of perpetration.

A perpetrator can cause trauma indirectly, unconsciously, and accidentally. For example:

- Traumatised mothers or fathers do not consciously want to traumatise their children, but their behaviour may do so.
- A person who does not recognise his own traumatisation will likely unintentionally create new trauma situations through his romantic pursuits.
- Even someone who, when driving, accidentally hits a child becomes a perpetrator. He or she will potentially have to deal with the consequences of this perpetration for the rest of his/her life.
- When politicians issue decrees, the implementation by the police and the judicial system can lead to severe damage for millions of people.
- Large institutions like, for instance, the International Monetary Fund (IMF), can cause starvation through their financial policies.
- If someone gives orders to shoot and kill, he kills and traumatises indirectly. Warmongers and intellectual instigators who create images of the 'enemy' and encourage aggression in others are indirect trauma perpetrators.

Some trauma perpetrators respect no boundaries, neither legal nor moral ones. They may do things that are completely alien to any common moral sense, such as the rape of babies, years of sexual intercourse with their own daughter, attacking a wife with a knife, poisoning of public drinking fountains, torture, incinerating people in gas ovens, dropping of atomic bombs, and so on.

Being the victim

If someone has become a victim it is a fact; it has happened and cannot be reversed. When becoming a victim also results in them being traumatised, it means that they have experienced extreme fear of death and abandonment. Tremendous feelings of pain, fear, anger, shame, and disgust have developed within them. The moment of traumatisation means that they have reached a state of numbness in order to survive, in which their vital functions had to be extremely reduced.

Someone can only survive becoming a victim by suppressing and splitting off the traumatising experience and feelings. The greater the damage, the greater the mechanism for suppression that trauma victims have to develop in order to survive. However, to start with the good news: parts of the trauma victim's psyche remain healthy despite the trauma. The basic principle of the human psyche, as we have seen above, is to provide a person with clear access to the reality of the external world and within himself, and this is not completely destroyed by trauma. The reality principle of the human psyche can only be modified and restricted in relation to certain areas of reality, namely those connected with the trauma. This applies in particular to the relationship with the trauma perpetrator(s).

As long as a person cannot dissolve his victim mentality and his relationship with the perpetrator, the initially external terror of the trauma event now continues to exist within his being. That requires him to develop long-term and extremely strong trauma survival strategies. In the context of perpetrator-victim dynamics I call these survival strategies the 'victim-attitudes'. Figure 6 outlines the basic schema of the internal situation of a trauma victim.

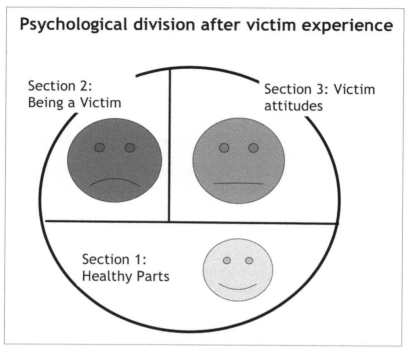

Figure 6: Psychological division of people with traumatising
victim experiences

Victim-attitudes as trauma survival strategies

If feeling like the trauma victim is to be avoided, victim-attitudes
as trauma survival strategies are required as long as the existential dependence on the perpetrator or perpetrators exists; these
strategies will actually ensure survival.

For example, if a soldier is threatened with execution if he
refuses to shoot the 'enemy', he has no other choice but to become
a murderer, even if the supposed enemy is in reality his friend or
companion. Other examples: Someone who otherwise has no
money to feed himself and his family cannot contradict his boss,
and has to follow their instructions, even if these are to his own
detriment. Someone in a couple relationship, who is scared of

being killed or harmed by his or her partner if they do not meet the partner's survival strategy demands, is forced to submit. Someone who in childhood cannot revolt against her parents has to find submissive ways to manage in order not to be destroyed.

The following are examples of trauma-victim-attitudes:

- denying being a victim and any associated feelings: "I am not afraid!" "I feel no anger." "I am fine here." "I lack nothing." "Everything is fine." "My husband has his good sides, too." "I had a happy childhood and I am grateful to my parents." "The important thing is that I have a job." "I like being German/American/Russian ..." "Wars are normal."
- clenching the teeth and wanting to be strong: "Nothing can shake me easily!" "Survival of the fittest!" "I can cope with it!" "Big boys don't cry!" "I have an iron will!" "What does not kill me makes me stronger!"
- repressing memories about being a victim: "That is a long time ago." "I don't want to think back to my childhood." "I have long forgotten all of that." "That is only the past!" "I have handled that myself." "Things have to go on after all. I only look forward!"
- despising 'weakness' within themselves and others: "Grit your teeth and get over it". "Don't let yourself down!" "Don't be so emotional and whiny!" "I hate it when I am weak!" "I am not a cry-baby!" "This constant sentimentalism!" "Leave me alone with your constant psycho talk!" "You are a softy and a wimp!" "Social sponger!" "Not long to retirement!"
- blaming themselves for the harm suffered: "It's my own fault." "I was a naughty child." "I never really paid attention." "I provoked my husband." "I should have kept my mouth shut!" "I was leaning too far out of the window in my job." "I always get everything wrong!"
- feeling ashamed about the harm suffered: "I am embarrassed!" "I am bad." "I am ashamed about that." "I am stupid and ugly!" "I am worthless."

- considering damage as fair punishment for their neediness, carelessness, and their existence: "I deserved the beating, because I was cheeky." "I should have made more of an effort." "I always want too much." "I also felt some pleasure whilst being raped." "I have to learn to be more humble."

When a trauma victim cannot entirely deny the damage she has suffered, she usually assumes responsibility for what has happened, and functions under the illusion that the right conduct and the right attitude would offer protection from further and new damage. Therefore, she is constantly focused on the perpetrator. In fact it seems then best not even to perceive and describe the perpetrator as such, but instead to assume the perpetrator's viewpoint and identify with their needs. What does this person need and want? What can I do for them so that they are more satisfied with me in the future? How can I make them happy? How can I better serve my parents, my company, my country, my faith? What do others need from me? The act of identifying and sympathizing with the needs of the perpetrator is often called "The Stockholm Syndrome" after events that happened during the hostage taking at a Swedish bank in 1973.

The trauma victim actually has to defend the perpetrator, for example through the following statements: "Should someone call XY a perpetrator and speak ill of him (or her) I have to defend him. If it comes to a possible legal prosecution, I have to defend him and claim his innocence. I need him and he needs me. We have to make a stand against everything that causes him difficulties and could split us up. If necessary, I would even commit perjury. That is how I make myself indispensable to him. He is nothing without me and I am nothing without him. Besides, I owe him so much: my life, my work, and my national identity. I know he is not perfect and makes mistakes, too. However, I have a big heart and can forgive that. To understand everything is to forgive everything! Surely, my love and affection can turn him into a better person and discourage him from committing more crimes. At least he deserves another chance. He needs me for that."

Victims who identify with the perpetrator show an 'addiction to harmony'. The relationship must not come into conflict, whether it is a political party, a company, a marriage, or a family, or at least nothing private should escape to the outside world. Criticism of circumstances and behaviours of individuals is perceived as threatening and will be ignored as long as possible. Those who possibly complain about being a victim have to be warned to be humble, and silenced.

This in the end leads trauma victims to feel personally responsible for the whole world. They have to be particularly peaceful, consume as little as possible, always help when others are in need, and always be willing to forgive and forget. They take care of those wounded in wars, look after refugees, comfort the injured, and clear away the corpses that the perpetrators produce.

People with a victim attitude are overly anxious and overly adjusted. They tend to be submissive, passive, and forbearing, suffering in silence. If they complain or occasionally lament their situation, they do so without looking at the real causes. They do not like others to point out the real reasons for their plight and that of other trauma victims. They only seek recognition for their immense ability to suffer and their unshakable submissiveness. They expect nothing more than perhaps a few words of encouragement from a person of authority.

"Those who do not work ...

... should not eat!" I probably absorbed this key phrase of the fascist ideology in Nazi Germany through my mother's milk. My mother only breastfed me for a few weeks after I was born. "I didn't have much myself!" was her reasoning. She was the sixth of nine children from a poor peasant family and throughout her life, she could not let go of the experiences of her deprived childhood. Every coin she turned twice before it was spent with a guilty conscience.

Additionally, my grandmother, my mother's mother, confessed to me that she had not wanted to have children with her husband, my grandfather. She had had to marry him although she had wanted to marry someone else.

After my abrupt weaning from breast-feeding, the feeding with milk powder nearly cost me my life. If the family doctor had not noticed that I was losing weight rather than gaining it and made my parents feed me on rice gruel I would have not survived the first year of my life.

I grew up in a working class household, and that meant that there was only money paid for hours actually worked, or for a specific amount of contracted work. The former was the case with my father and his hourly pay in the quarry, and the latter was for the work my mother accepted at home. She, my sister, and I had to sacrifice holidays so she could plait hundreds of badges for the uniforms of soldiers from the Federal Armed Forces, or paint grey plastic toy Indians with colour so that a little money came into the house. At least I was able to play with the big toy figures that were defective, and made myself popular with some friends.

At the village school that I went to, the parents of most of the children were farmers or workers. Even the village tailor was better off because he could sew the commissioned suits and coats in the warmth of his house. The pastor and the teacher at the school ruthlessly beat the pupils. Nevertheless, they received sausages and fresh meat free of charge from our parents if a pig was slaughtered in one of the houses. This was probably not so much an appreciation of their intellectual and pedagogical work but rather a kind of bribery and an expression of subservience.

The refugees, who came to our village after the Second World War, starving and helpless, were met with contempt by many of the local people. For a long time it was not clear to me that my father, too, was a 'refugee'; the Sudeten Germans considered themselves displaced. Since my father was a shepherd until I was six years old, I was only known in our village as the "Schafferle" – the son of the shepherd.

At my grammar school I was ashamed to reveal my father's job in front of the class; however this was printed in the school journals every year as 'worker'. The other children were able to state their parents as teachers or bankers. Here was a socially widespread victim attitude that I took on: "Shame on you because you are poor! If you are poor, you are to blame because you have not learned anything. If you have not learned anything, you are stupid. And then you have to do the dirty work that nobody else wants to do voluntarily."

As soon as I was 16, I worked during the long summer holidays in order to earn my own money. At that time, my schoolmates from elementary school had already started apprenticeships, and received a trainee salary, so they were no longer fully financially dependent on their parents. Some of them were even able to afford a brand new motorcycle with their wages, and could take the village girls on the rear seat to the discothèque on Saturday evenings. My holiday job income was only enough for an old, unfashionable Kreidler motorbike with a lame 3.2hp, which even after a trendy paint job was not very impressive. At least I was mobile and did not have to get up so early anymore to catch the school bus into town.

My first holiday job, a four-week period, was in construction, and during the subsequent summer holidays, I worked in a marble factory. This showed me the reality of my mother's words: "If you refuse to learn at school then you will have to work in the quarry like your father!" The quarry was a much tougher job than construction, in which sanded and polished marble was relocated into buildings. Breaking stones outdoors where giant blocks of stone were crushed was much more daunting than the marble factory. But here it was terribly loud and permanently damp because of the water needed to cut and grind the stones. Nevertheless, at least there was a roof over my head and I was not exposed to the weather elements. Even though there were health risks because of the dust and chemicals used to patch up holes in the blocks, at least there was no risk of being killed from blowing up stone blocks or of sliding into the bottom of the quarry.

As a small boy, I was glad every evening when I saw the bus that transported my father home from work. Once again I thought he had avoided death, unlike our neighbour who had been crushed by a heavy stone whilst loading them onto a truck. In addition, especially because my mother's father had been struck dead by a falling branch during forestry work before I was born, I was in constant fear of lethal accidents.

So I studied for better grades, and later I was surprised at the amount of money one could make even though nothing substantial seemed to have been achieved at the end of the day. No heavy loads had to be moved, no exhaustion of the body was needed. It was just sitting in meetings, drinking coffee, maybe reading a scientific article, and writing a couple of pages of text the whole day. Or, as a researcher, to observe other people with their laborious and dangerous employment, question them briefly about their activity, and then encode the results on complicated questionnaires back at the office.

The connection between performance and wages remained a mystery to me as a child, teenager, and long into my adult working life. In accordance with my primary victim attitude "You don't get to eat if you have not worked hard", I always had a guilty conscience, wondering if I had really performed well enough for the money I received from my employer. Even during my holiday work I had always suspiciously observed others and judged them as to whether they had really done their duties or were just lazy.

Only much later did I realise that there is no correlation between a certain amount of money and what had actually been achieved during a day. After all, I questioned, how could the quality of a work activity be harmonised with the quantity of a sum of money? Wages are, despite contractual standards and calculations, one component of a macro-social employment system. Wages are calculated according to the number of those willing to work, and those who are unemployed and are prepared to earn the lowest possible hourly rates. This is so that the 'suppliers of work', employers who are actually taking other people's work, can make a financial profit. In the German language the distortion between "Arbeitnehmer" = 'employee' and "Arbeitgeber" = 'employer' conveys in an almost classical way the ideology of perpetrator-victim reversal in the capitalistic economy.

My father was never interested in my critical objections to this kind of economy. He was glad to have his work, and spent part of his wages with the activity of breeding chickens and pigeons. He had little interest in protest and was quick to refer to Adolph Hitler, who would have sent today's work-shy riffraff packing to labour camps.

Today I am relatively well off, and yet I still work a lot because I enjoy what I do, and consider my work to be meaningful. At a recent visit to my bank I told the banking advisor, who was trying to sell me the most lucrative investments, "I am already rich enough. I have enough money for my modest daily needs. Moreover, I am uncomfortable with the idea of taking part in the exploitation of other people through stock and real estate funds, or to commission 'finance experts' to speculate with my money – including the risk of incurring great losses."

"Let your money work for you" – a casually uttered ideology that veils the perpetrator-victim dynamics of a competitive market economy. Today the shares of armaments manufacturers are particularly lucrative. Should I take my bit of money and get involved in the big business of war?

Now and then I come across money issues during therapy, for instance if a client who is a doctor with a successful surgery suffers from existential fears. A closer look reveals that these existential fears originally stem from his traumatising childhood. These feelings disappear as soon as this person can feel the existential terror of his childhood.

A patient who worked in an investment bank was completely focused on doing bigger and bigger financial transactions. This he intended to distract him from the fact that as a child his father had left him with a traumatised mother, who constantly threatened to commit suicide, until she finally actually did kill herself.

In my experience many people's careers function as trauma-survival strategies, the psychotherapist's included, of course! Only someone who has seen this can really start looking for a truly worthwhile economic activity that is good for them and through which they can bring about something beneficial for others.

People who are not in touch with themselves continue to lose themselves in the work that they do, and they allow others to abuse them for other purposes. They let their personal integrity and moral standards be bought and compromised with money, not even noticing when they cause harm to others through their actions, turning into perpetrators themselves and accomplices to other perpetrators. They ignore their responsibility for their professional conduct. To oppose the collective ideologies is frightening. The traumatized collective can become merciless towards the individual who does not share their ideas and motives, which are regarded as normal and reasonable (Harrari, 2017, S 202 ff.).

Victim identity

The life purpose of the trauma victim becomes the controlled social interactions with perpetrators. Almost all of their vital energy flows into this programme of survival; it becomes their mission in life. Even if dependence on the perpetrator no longer actually exists, or the trauma perpetrator is no longer alive, many trauma victims are unable to stop this programme of survival within them.

They cannot psychologically leave the relationship with their perpetrator because over the years they have deeply internalised the perpetrator into their psychological structures and suppressed themselves even further. The connection with the perpetrator was the only way in which they could emotionally feel a bit livelier and not completely alone and abandoned.

Often the child cares for their perpetrator mother and father with great devotion until their death. Even after their death, a great deal of commitment is given to the maintenance of the graves. Even sexually traumatised children as adults defend their perpetrators if the 'scandal of the abuse' is made public. Traumatised war veterans will not speak ill about the government that with lies and extensive propaganda took them into war. Instead, they are happy when they are honoured with medals for their 'services to people and country'. People who have developed a victim identity as their survival strategy show a fatalistic resignation: "Men/women are just the way they are. That will never change!"

As long as he do not consciously want to give up his relationship with the trauma perpetrator, the victim stays attached to him or her. Only if trauma victims systematically work on their repressed and denied psychological pain, and focus on processing their fears will they be able to successfully exit their relationship with the perpetrator. That can be a long and painstaking process. First, it requires that they claim back their identity and their will.

Psychology uses several terms to characterize perpetrator-victim relationships (Huber et al, 2013; Peichl, 2007; Vogt, 2012):

- *Perpetrator identification:* The victim assumes the attitudes and behaviour patterns of the perpetrator, and goes against her own interests, even when the perpetrator is not present. The 'I' of the perpetrator rules in the psyche of the trauma victims, instead of their own 'I'.
- *Perpetrator loyalty:* The victim is loyal to the perpetrator, gives priority to the perpetrator's interests, and defends him from attacks.
- *Perpetrator introjects:* The actions of the perpetrator sear into the psyche of the victim to the point of being entirely at the mercy of him. The victim vividly senses and feels the perpetrator within herself, and finds it difficult to gain any distance from him. That is especially the case when the perpetrator connects their perpetration of the victim with their own idea of themselves as the saviour of the victim: "I am hitting you for your own good, because I am the only person that really loves you"; "Without me you would be nothing!"

Now it is clear to me why I repeatedly went from my victim identity into bullying processes at school, as well as in my work life. The fact that I had not been wanted as a child created in me a fundamental lifelong guilt: Because I exist, I am responsible for my mother's misfortunes. Therefore, I have to prove myself as both thankful and useful, but in addition, I will never be able to pay off my debt as long as I continue to exist. This situation of being unwanted in my mother's womb kept repeating itself in my biography: one minute I am there, alive and full of vitality and drive, the next minute I receive a dampener, a 'no' to my existence from others (my mother): "You should not be here!"

This happened to me most strongly when I was newly appointed as a lecturer at university, and some of my female colleagues and female students rejected me from a feminist perspective because I was a man and not the woman they had wished for as their colleague. This continued later when I wanted to introduce constellations work at the university, as I considered it a brilliant method for conveying psychological knowledge in a practical and clear way. Again came a vehement 'no' from others, that put a huge damper on my vitality and desire to explore.

As a result of work that I did for myself afterwards concerning this bullying situation, I now know that the scared and very early split off part of myself offered an ideal target for others to work off their frustration and jealousy, and to boost their own image. I was always on the defensive, and could not retaliate since my perception was that it was my fault when others suffered because of my presence. Even though I was able to get angry, and even show a little rage now and again, I was defenceless, since at that time I had not yet met my original trauma and my own trauma feelings. Therefore, I could not leave and had to endure the hostility of others, because it re-evoked my experience at that early age: to leave my mother's womb would have meant to die.

From trauma victim to perpetrator

People are not always comfortable in their trauma-victim attitudes. They may express their suppressed anger and endless pain, built up over the years, in concealed verbal, and sometimes in outright, aggression. However, this happens primarily in the presence of people that they consider to be weaker than themselves, rather than towards the perpetrator. Preferred objects of such hatred and aggression will be other trauma victims, that the person perceives as people who possibly take advantage of their status as an officially acknowledged victim, (for example, asylum seekers, the unemployed, and welfare recipients). Those victims in fact are innocents who have had nothing to do with the original cause of the person's plight and anger. This can create a classic chain of aggression: a man beats a woman; the woman beats the eldest child; this child maltreats the younger sibling, who kicks the cat. Then people freely become enraged about the alleged social scroungers, or those foreigners they consider inferior to themselves. They feel that their nationality is a sign of their personal quality, automatically elevating them above anyone who does not possess their nationality.

Self-destructive behaviours are also common victim attitudes: denying one's basic needs such as sufficient food and sleep, and enacting self-harm by smoking. There is an absence of a healthy 'I' to intervene in such situations, and with young girls, these behaviours can become obsessive and compulsive. Their trauma-survival strategies take such a severe form of self-hatred, which they can no longer control. Some may even go so far as to try to swallow razor blades.

The worse the victim's trauma experiences, and the greater their dependence on the perpetrator, the more harmful the forms of victim attitude survival strategies become. These include all forms of addiction and drug dependence, refusal to eat ('anorexia'), compulsive overeating and vomiting ('bulimia'), or without vomiting afterwards ('obesity' and 'adiposity').

Suffering from pain can be experienced as a short-term release from a permanent inner tension. Pain is overcome by further pain, and the masochist victim looks for a sadistic sexual perpetrator as a saviour.

Victim attitudes can also manifest in chronic physical illnesses (for example diabetes, rheumatism, stomach ulcers, cancer) (Ruppert & Banzhaf, 2017). The transformation of an early trauma event related to a perpetrator-victim relationship into a 'disease' that seems biological, actually comes from the fact that the victim is stuck in a perpetrator-victim relationship. This transformation into an illness also relies on the helping systems of traumatised societies that actively support this victim attitude. These healthcare and welfare systems then collectively deny the existence of any perpetrator-victim relationships. The traces of the perpetrator-victim issue, made visible through the physical suffering, is ignored and blurred by the complexity of medical diagnoses, proposals for psychotherapeutic work for behavioural change, and socio-pedagogical offers of taking care.

It is no wonder, then, that such well-intentioned diagnoses and treatments result so often in 'chronic depression', the surrendering of our free will and the suppression of our own needs. This consequence is then either quietly accepted, fought with psychotropic drugs, or supplemented with acts of violence such as electroconvulsive therapy – a blast of electricity blown into the brain under the pseudo-scientific premise that this will remix their cocktail of hormones! The more one tries to escape into an victim identity, the greater the possibility that one becomes, in turn, a victim to medical, psychotherapeutic, and social work treatments, turning one into an ongoing experimental subject of the measures of those who impose their useless concepts of diagnoses and therapies, if necessary by force (Ruppert, 2002).

Thus, in the end many trauma victims resign, wishing they were dead. Suicidal thoughts and suicide attempts are themselves trauma-survival strategies, as paradoxical that may sound. Suicide appears the ultimate way out of the confrontation with the unbearable and shameful feelings of one's own victimhood. This resignation often started at the beginning of life, since the traumatised person might have had to survive an attempted abortion in the womb of his mother, or was seriously unwanted: suicide seems like a return to the starting point. Do I want to exist, when originally I was not welcomed?

Victim attitudes as collective trauma-survival strategies

Victim attitudes as trauma-survival strategies are widespread in traumatised societies. In fact these behaviours are seen as culturally normal. Often over many generations it is simply about enduring, surviving, and functioning in a variety of situations. This means that traumatised societies have a stubborn adherence to old traditions and values, such as to their religion, ancestor worship or death cults. The particular national history is invoked repeatedly, even if it is not much more than a series of wars with neighbouring states and violent conflicts within their society.

Through education, history lessons, indoctrination, and mystical rituals every new generation is burdened by the suffering and traumas of previous generations, supported by the argument that they have to stick to their roots and not renounce their origins.

Scientific rationalisations, which blank out psychological realities as irrelevant, allow a traumatised society to avoid confrontation with the massive facts of endemic psychotraumas, perpetration and victimisation. Even terrorism in a traumatised society is in the end not more than a trauma-survival strategy. It follows a programme of self-sacrifice for the nation, religion, and/or family as can be seen as an example within the Palestinian youth. A family clan expects that their child will blow himself up with a body belt full of explosives in service to their society, even though it is known and obvious that this will cause further violence from Israel, a state that can be certain of continued military and economic support from America (Chomsky, 2016). The more a person has had to surrender to being a victim, and has had to disappear from himself, the more he/she will cling onto a collective construct as a substitute for self, his only raison d'être: my nation, my state, my faith!

Being a Perpetrator

Being a trauma perpetrator is a lasting fact. If someone inflicts harm on another person that he cannot make up for, and that is psychologically unacceptable, it becomes a traumatising life experience, not just for the victim, but also for the perpetrator, leading to permanent damage to the psyche. As long as the person's psyche can function in a healthy way – every

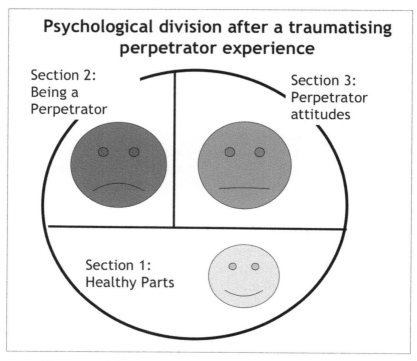

Figure 7: Division of a human psyche after a traumatising perpetrator experience

perpetrator will have some residual healthy psyche – the perpetrator will have a nagging guilty conscience about the reality of what he has done. He feels guilty and ashamed, and he may be afraid of being socially ostracised. These are stressful emotional conditions that are also unbearable, and so these feelings have to be split off.

So perpetrators, like their victims, have to psychologically split in order to survive, even more so if they continue to live in the same community (e.g. family) with their victims and relatives of the victim. Figure 7 represents this situation.

Therefore, to function through perpetrator attitudes is the trauma-survival strategy of a perpetrator. These perpetrator attitudes can vary widely, principally serving to expunge feelings of fear, guilt, and shame from the conscious experience of the perpetrator.

Perpetrator attitudes

Should it not be completely possible to hide their own offence, trauma perpetrators try to play down the damage they have caused the victim. To this end, parents often say to their children such things as: "There's no reason to cry!" "That wasn't so bad!" "It was just a slap on the bottom!" "It hurts me much more than it hurts you." "I'm doing this for your own good." "You will thank me one day." "We never used to do you any harm!" "You can't make an omelette without breaking eggs." "That's normal!" "I'm much worse off than you!" "If only my childhood had been as good as yours!" "The things we've done for you and then you're ungrateful and reproach us!" Thus, the victim has to remain silent, and if he do not he is silenced with further traumatisation.

Perpetrators learn to appease and talk to the point where what they have done is completely diminished. Another strategy that a perpetrator will use is to shift attention to trivialities in order deflect from the main issue; even better if they can hide behind 'practical constraints'. For example "This war was unavoidable for the long-term safeguarding of peace." Or "We have to increase the pace of work and reduce wages to keep us surviving on the market and to safeguard the remaining jobs." Talk shows about controversial political and social topics are a good opportunity to study those perpetrator attitudes.

Trauma perpetrators develop high levels of skills in order to deflect from their responsibility, and to support their own interests, deeds and the consequences thereof. Even high-level Nazi activists pleaded at the end of their reign of terror that they had either "not known" the consequences of their actions, or were only "executing orders". A well-known example of this was Adolf Eichmann's behaviour at his trial in Israel. Another popular, and even at times legally accepted, excuse is being innocent of one's actions due to alcohol intoxication.

It is a relief for trauma perpetrators to be able to hide in a collective. "Nobody noticed anything and everybody just did his duty." "That was just the people at the top, we as people didn't know it. We were just doing our job."

When the perpetrator actions can no longer be denied, the main aim of the trauma perpetrator then becomes to portray himself as innocent. What is attempted at this stage is a 'perpetrator-victim reversal'; the perpetrator portrays himself or herself as the actual victim, spreading lies about the real victim, in order to accuse and embarrass them: "That child provoked me so much that I just lost my patience." "This woman/child seduced me." "If you are still poor you clearly haven't learned anything at school!" "We had to massively bomb Iraq because of Saddam Hussein's weapons of mass destruction." This is how victims become accused of being perpetrators. They are blamed and embarrassed when the real perpetrator's harmful intentions are projected onto the victims, so that the actual perpetrators no longer have to feel afraid of retribution; they would be legally entitled to protection – with force if necessary, because morality and the law would then be on their side. In this scenario victims who defend themselves against violence are portrayed as particularly nasty, devious, and dangerous and they have to be all the more severely punished.

The perpetrator-victim reversal is particularly apparent when dealing with so-called 'refugees'. These people, who are very clearly the victims of military and economic wars, are portrayed as perpetrators if they seek refuge in a country that originated the wars or supports the wars. The real culprits who lead to this flight and displacement are never directly named in the debates over 'the flood of refugees' and 'admission quotas'.

In order to distract from their guilty consciences, perpetrators make a great effort to demonstrate a clear conscience in the public eye. They like to present themselves as great humanitarians, presenting their wars as peacekeeping missions, referring to the many jobs they have created, their tireless work for the common good or their generous donations for humanitarian purposes and scientific research.

They adorn themselves with honorary leadership of charitable organisations or even found charities themselves. From my therapeutic work, I know of perpetrators who sexually traumatised children and at the same time credibly and convincingly acted piously in church and decorated the altar.

Because perpetrators cannot show their true 'I', this having been buried so deeply inside them in the course of their trauma biography, they have to strive for a pseudo-identity. That is only possible through making a distinction between themselves and others based on, "I am not like. . ." Their own self does not exist. Whatever a perpetrator chooses as a substitute for his identity remains a façade behind which he hides. Most popular with perpetrators is the descent into a 'we': "we Germans", "we Americans", "we Russians", "we Christians", "we Muslims" etc. In this way, perpetrators can continue their activities without interference. After all, what they do is in fact no longer for their own sake but in the service of a supposedly common cause, and so nationalism, religious fanaticism, and chauvinism are popular and widespread amongst trauma perpetrators. They do what they do with a good conscience.

Because they do not know their own self, and have no independent way of defining themselves, trauma perpetrators continue to need the relationship with the victims and cannot leave them alone. Trauma perpetrators are manically fixated on their victims. They forcefully attribute all their own bad intentions and deeds onto their victims. When, for instance 'the communists' ceased to be the enemy of the moment they had to be replaced by the next scapegoat – 'the foreigners' or 'the Muslims'. Without victims, trauma perpetrators are nothing – just an empty shell. If we consider how trauma victims are often obsessively concerned about their perpetrators their entire life, then this realisation becomes absolutely shocking and sobering: in reality the trauma perpetrators are completely empty inside; all they are, is simply a façade.

Alongside the more defensive variety of perpetrator attitudes, there are also radically offensive ones: perpetrators who can be recognised by the speed and extremity of reaction they exhibit when they are being criticised – they are easily offended, acting appalled, hurt, and deeply insulted. They try to put the blame for their exaggerated suffering onto their critics and conversely shame them, ridiculing and abusing those who dare criticise them as if they were the greatest possible villains in all humanity. For example, Adolf Hitler started in 1937 to regard the Sudeten Germans, who lived outside of Germany, as citizens of his Reich. With the military invasion of Prague, on the 15th March 1939, he broke up the Czechoslovakian Republic and assimilated it into his project of the 'Greater German Reich'. In 2017, the Turkish president Tayyip Erdogan called the German chancellor Angela Merkel a Nazi, and likened her to Adolf Hitler. With that, he reclaimed the emigrated Turks in Germany as his people. From now on, they should have access to the best schools, live in the most beautiful houses, and quickly reproduce. Every Turkish woman should ideally have five children. He promised his supporters that soon Europe would be dominated by Turkish culture. Hitler did similar things with the German race.

Preventatively, so to speak, perpetrators demand respect, admiration and special treatment for themselves, preventing anyone from looking behind their 'wolf in sheep's clothing' mask.

Trauma perpetrators prefer to surround themselves with people who are submissive and admire them. That is why they attach a lot of importance to show, pomp and splendour, and a neat external appearance. With men, this is often smoothly parted hair, with a suit and tie; with women the make-up often cannot be applied thick enough. Royal garments, official robes and uniforms complete the look, so that a trauma perpetrator does not have to show himself as an ordinary human, but gives the impression of being someone very special, chosen from history, even close to divine.

Secrecy and looking away

Trauma perpetrators shy away from the public eye with their exploits, keeping their plans secret. They build a façade of normality around their secrets, trying to convince others that they do not have any. Some do this very skilfully, while others make it blatantly obvious that they lie and cheat. However, my own psyche has to be in a healthy condition in order for me to recognise that. If I am in a trauma survival state myself, it will be difficult for me to diagnose the lies of perpetrators as such, and not fall victim to them. Where perpetrator loyalty rules, blinded by trauma and supported by media propaganda, trauma perpetrators can get away with brazen lies (Wernicke, 2017).

Trauma perpetrators have it easy whenever surrounded by other traumatised people, especially when those people are in a victim attitude, as then the perpetrators can do almost anything they want to them. The perception of victims is so severely impeded, and they are so emotionally stunted, confused in their actions and unquestioningly obedient, that they are constantly prey to the whims of perpetrators They are emotionally stunted, act foolishly, and are unquestioningly obedient. Since they are afraid of the perpetrators, and often financially dependent on them, they look away and do not ask any questions.

In Austria a man who had already been sentenced for rape, was able to imprison his daughter in a basement shelter, and produce seven children with her. Three of those children he took out of the cell and put on his doorstep with a letter that he had extorted from his imprisoned daughter. For over 24 years nobody expressed any suspicion that something might not be right; not his wife, not the other children from the relationship between him and his wife, not the 100 tenants who stayed in the same house during that time, not the authorities, not his friends. When we are in our surviving mode, the elephant in our own living room cannot be seen no matter how big he is.

Amongst themselves, trauma perpetrators are like feuding brothers. They stake out their claims of control, form alliances and leave each other alone as long as they do not get in each other's way. 'Dog does not eat dog.' However, because of their own hidden inner life, they have an acute sense for picking up if another perpetrator is concealing secrets, or is lying or cheating. They take advantage of this sense in order to blackmail other perpetrators, if it promises to be to their advantage. Trauma perpetrators, amongst themselves, can give the impression of being the closest of friends, but if one perpetrator somehow gets in the way of another, this friendship can quickly turn into relentless hostility. If personal interests of power and profit demand it, the former 'friend' is sacrificed with nothing more than a shrug of the shoulders. Therefore, perpetrators do not trust anyone, and are deeply suspicious people. For example, Stalin's growing paranoia became increasingly apparent towards the end of his life. He killed the witnesses to his own murderous actions.

Perpetrator ideologies

The ideal situation for perpetrators is that they can justify their actions as being in the service of the community, and present their behaviour as something good. For this a political, economic, religious, or simply inter-familial ideology is called for that can justify acts of war, exploitation, murder and torment of people, or the torture of their own children or partners as good and reasonable. In this way, victims are not just damaged and traumatised, but they can also be despised and mocked – for example because of the colour of their skin, their gender, their nationality, their religion, their alleged lack of education or their mental or physical disabilities. They can then be treated as objects without any bad conscience, like scum rather than as human subjects. Therefore, trauma perpetrators depersonalise their victims as much as possible by various means, such as dress codes (uniforms, headscarves), obligations of conduct (eating, praying, style of hair and beard), name-calling, numbering (prisoner's numbers) and labelling (diagnoses like 'schizophrenia'). Perpetrators want individuals only to be able to perceive themselves in the context of the whole system. This is supported by the fact that trauma victims often seek salvation by disappearing into a crowd so as not to attract any attention, and then through the anonymity of the crowd, they can then express their own perpetrator attitudes ("We are the people!").

Essentially, perpetrator ideologies exist so as to divide groups of people by creating and cultivating images of an enemy: 'the Jews', 'the Muslims', 'the Fat Cats', 'the benefit scroungers', 'the establishment', 'the lying press', 'the capitalists', 'the asylum seekers', 'the homosexuals', 'the terrorists', 'the communists', 'the negroes', 'the redskins', 'the slit-eyes', 'the women', 'the men' and so on ...

When the Soviet Union still existed as an alternative political system, the term 'communist' was extensively used in the west to randomly discredit and politically silence anyone who opposed. For the colonialists of the 18th to 20th centuries a 'negro' was a subhuman whose enslavement was not considered a sin in the eyes of God. Independent of their tribal affiliation and their diverse physical appearances, all indigenous people were classed as semi-savages and it was permitted for the immigrant conquerors of the American continent to shoot them. Calling the Viet Cong 'slit-eyes' during the Vietnam War, for example, made it clear for US soldiers who the enemy was.

In Germany, after the fall of the Nazi dictatorship, the most effective way to outlaw someone politically or scientifically is to brand him or her either as an 'extreme right-winger' or a 'left-wing conspiracy theorist'. According to their historical context, every country has its own way of labelling and defaming its critics, and in so doing exposing their own perpetrator nature. Whilst the Holocaust was justified by the National Socialists with the stance that the 'Jews' were the enemy of the German people, after World War II anyone in Germany who dared to criticise the aggressive settlement policy of the Israeli State in Palestine was declared 'anti-Semitic'. The Turkish President Erdogan, by calling all his opponents terrorists, exploited the globally acceptable argument of labelling political enemies as 'terrorists'.

Male claims of dominance have been justified for hundreds of years by reasoning that women are unable to think rationally and incapable of controlling their sexual desires. What better way to illustrate the phenomenon of perpetrator-victim reversal: a man is allowed to act out his sexual cravings on a woman, since she is only a thoughtless and dishonourable whore. Conversely, some women, in their victim attitude, interpret this male claim of dominance as protection, even seeing it as a noble action by the man. In this way, the male perpetrator tendency towards assault becomes reinterpreted as a form of protection for the woman against unwanted attention from other males. Therefore, whilst perpetrating, the perpetrator appears to be, at the same time, the saviour of their victim.

It is true that the majority of violent criminals are male, and men make up 95% of the prisons population. But what is difficult to accept, especially for 'feminists', is the idea of the traumatised mother who, based on her own victim attitude, traumatises her children because her lack of a sense of self impedes her ability to love and relate to others.

As an example, in a resonance process, the resonator for a mother, when questioned by her daughter (the client) came up with this memorable sentence: "You owe me your life!" This fell on fertile ground with the daughter, who was still attached to the ideology that she owed her life to her mother.

In this way, traumatised mothers unconsciously and unintentionally bring the next generation of traumatised men into the world and raise them to have marked perpetrator attitudes. With the topic of female circumcision, too, it is almost exclusively mothers and grandmothers, who inflict this cruelty on their female children and grandchildren. And in patriarchal families it is the mothers who enforce and feed their daughters' victim attitudes and their sons' perpetrator attitudes.

Perpetrator identity

Just as with victim attitudes, the perpetrator attitudes also radicalise further over time. Perpetrators behave as though they were completely without fear, and nothing and nobody can stop them. If trauma perpetrators succeed in convincing themselves and others of their perpetrator ideology, they have less and less need to conceal their actions, and can act out completely pointless and exhaustive violence. In this way, violence is always justified against a specified enemy. "The only good Indian is a dead one" white settlers said during the conquest of the American continent. Today though, many would still agree when it is said that all forms of terror may be employed in order to kill terrorists. The drone campaign against terrorism, initiated by the American President Barack Obama, terrorized the entire civilian population in states such as Afghanistan, Yemen, and Iraq. However, the influence of Barack Obama's governance is still well recognised in most other countries.

Perpetrators can even feel lust, feelings of triumph, or pride when causing violence and destruction: "I really nailed that whore ...!" The social psychologist Harald Welzer analysed the wiretap transcripts of the Allies in World War II and discovered the level of enthusiasm and pleasure with which, for instance, pilots in the German dive-bombers hunted defenceless victims (Welzer, 2011).

Perpetrators do not think of themselves as perpetrators; in fact, they are often proud of their acts of perpetration. Since they project their split off trauma feelings outwardly, they claim that the evil that actually exists inside them, exists solely in the outside world. Freed from social inhibitions, trauma perpetrators are in such perpetual need that they must continually create new situations in order to convince themselves, and everyone else, that all people feel threatened by this 'evil', not just them. Compassion for these 'sinister forces' would be a sign of weakness, which would have to be overcome internally. In the end, they convince themselves that their perpetrator existence and actions are the only possible ways to save the world from 'the powers of darkness'. The American Ex-President Ronald Reagan called the Soviet Union an 'empire of evil' in a speech on the 8th March 1983.

To establish peace with increasingly deadly weapons is the

absurd but logical consequence of this perpetrator attitude. Out of this mindset, secret societies develop, which are a crude fraternisation of people from military, economic, and religious elites. These secret societies then spawn aggressive secret services, and even such groupings as satanic cults that in their psychological confusion and emotional numbness worship evil, seeing it as the actual good, even sacrificing their babies and children to it (Huber, 1998, Hahn, 2016).

Even the chief ideologues of an 'Islamic State' are only following the logical consequence of something already established in their perpetrator attitudes from the beginning: 'We are the only true believers and we have the right to behead all nonbelievers'. Their religion gives them the justification for every possible cruelty. The reasoning of trauma perpetrators moves in abstract, mythological images, consisting of false claims and logical contradictions; Hitler's book 'Mein Kampf' bears testimony to this, as does the 'manifesto' of the Norwegian mass murderer Anders B. Breivik. Even though trauma perpetrators are sometimes very sly and clever, they are also mentally very confused. They do not understand that their sole endeavour is the endless fighting of trauma with trauma.

Trauma perpetrators in power

If perpetrator-victim dynamics, with their complex interactions, are not recognised and discussed in a community, be it a country or a political, economical or cultural institution, no dialogue can progress beyond a black and white form of thinking; everything ends up being reduced to a simple schema of good & evil. Therefore, red lines are drawn depending on the current interests of the powerful and rich: on one side are the 'good', on the other are the 'bad'. Whole societies are polarised and split, and solidarity cannot be sustained. Anyone who, despite much encouragement and plenty of propaganda, still has not decided to cheer for the 'good' side (for the trauma perpetrators), is likely to be seen as one of the 'bad' side, and then forced to suffer their fate.

In the name of a supposed higher set of values such as 'the

fatherland', 'the empire', 'this grand nation of ours', 'Islam', 'Christianity' and 'family honour,' even the most inhumane acts can be experienced as a community's blessing. Anyone who kills in the name of these unquestioned 'higher values' is not a murderer or terrorist, but a hero and a freedom fighter, and so he doesn't deserve punishment or contempt, but instead fame, medals, awards, or the promise of eternal life in 'paradise', because he has performed a great service to the 'common good.'

Trauma perpetrators believe that they must, and can, save the community, whether a family, a village or a whole nation. Family clans, for example, may set up criminal networks, like the Mafia. If trauma perpetrators succeed in getting into a position of power, they can silence, imprison, or destroy anyone who criticises them or questions their actions. Therefore, trauma perpetrators strive for total control; everything must be subject to their will: the police, the legal system, the military and the media; all are actually kept in their job by the actions of the perpetrator, because perpetrators make many enemies. As politicians trauma perpetrators end up as dictators striving for total control over their trauma victims, they need everything in the state to run according to their thinking and their perpetrator logic and behaviour. Then there is no limit to the cruel ideas within themselves and their accomplices for the execution of their insanity.

The slaughter of thousands of Jews by the German Fascists in the Third Reich (1933-45) was actually not easy to justify and cope with psychologically. Heinrich Himmler admitted this in his convoluted speech to officers of the Wehrmacht in Posen on the 4th October 1943: "To have endured this and – apart for some exceptions of human weakness – to have remained decent has made us strong." The entire speech offers superb illustrative material for classical perpetrator attitudes.[4]

---

4   https://de.wikipedia.org/wiki/Posener_Reden

The accomplices

Perpetrators need accomplices, therefore they create a system of dependent people around them who will look away, or trivialise the perpetration, because they are relieved not to be in the victim role themselves. They will happily take advantage of all the privileges offered by the trauma perpetrator, and ally with him and identify with his attitudes. As journalists, professors, intellectuals, drinking companions, and as siblings, they will, each in their own way, justify and legitimise what the trauma perpetrators are doing. They become the intellectual mouthpieces of the perpetrators, spearheading their ideas, or simply allowing the perpetration to continue unquestioned.

What do perpetrators of trauma get out of it?

What do trauma perpetrators get out of investing their vital energy, intelligence and their money in being perpetrators? How do they benefit from their actions when they win one battle and then start the next? Their victories in war produce traumatised soldiers and civilians, so what do they gain from ruling a traumatised people? Their exploitative economic successes create an impoverished and sick society, so what do they get out of being surrounded by the resulting misery and hardship? What do they get out of their acts of rape and abuse as their traumatised partners become incapable of being in a relationship with them, and are no longer able to be good (sexual) partners? And perpetrator mothers and fathers – what do they get out of hitting their children and keeping them small and frightened? The result is that their traumatised children will cling on to them with their problems for their whole lives.

Unfortunately, the blindness to reality that trauma perpetrators suffer knows no limits. They may even construct bunkers deep in the ground with the idea of waging a nuclear war from there, the plan being to survive and afterwards to continue to rule the world. Apparently, trauma perpetrators would rather put up with the fallout of their actions than feel ashamed, or take actual responsibility for their misdeeds. They cannot feel the pain of their brutality because they do not feel themselves and have lost their own 'I'. If, therefore, they do not fall in one of their own battles, they will choose suicide rather than having to admit to failure and wrongdoing, as for example Hitler did.

To be perpetrator and victim all-in-one

Victims are crippled by fear and anxiety, and this blocks access to the left hemisphere of their brain, which then limits their ability to think and speak clearly (van der Kolk, 2014). Perpetrators, on the other hand, have to block out their fear and anxiety so that they can be perpetrators. The left hemisphere of their brain is then free to work in isolation from the right hemisphere, and so they are cut off from all feelings. In this way they are able to make cold calculations and use their logical intelligence without the limitations that compassion normally brings. Eventually perpetrators may even keep their fears numbed with the use of drugs in order to keep their perpetrator stance alive.

Threats of violence generally make a victim panic further and cripple them even more. Perpetrators, on the other hand, when faced with violence, are more likely to respond with violence themselves, since they are not in contact with their fear. Therefore, when two perpetrators come together their interactions can quickly escalate into violence, as each wants to outdo the other with demonstrations of fearlessness and propensity to violence. So they would then not even shy away from the use of nuclear weapons.

In reality, being a victim or a perpetrator rarely appears in the pure form. This is because the split off feelings of being a victim make him deaf and blind to the reality of the damage he is suffering, which is traumatising and causes psychological splits. The numbness towards himself turns into an insensitivity towards others. If someone is traumatised in the early stages of their life there is a danger, as already mentioned, that their entire life turns into a trauma biography.

Because of this, there is a strong likelihood that trauma victims will become trauma perpetrators, neither accepting being a victim nor being a perpetrator. Christian Pfeiffer, a German criminologist has found this connection confirmed again and again in his research on crime. In a report in the 'Süddeutsche Zeitung' from the 3rd January 2018, it is claimed: "The greatest common denominator amongst violent criminals statistically is that they were beaten in their childhood. Hundreds of studies indicate this. This biographical feature correlates most strongly with violent behaviour, more strongly than religion, origin, wealth, and education."[5]

This has many consequences as people oscillate between victim and perpetrator attitudes. Feelings of powerlessness and omnipotence surface alternately, unpredictable even to the person themselves.

Aggression and depression become the norm in everyday relationships of people who are imprisoned in their victim and perpetrator attitudes. On a stage for example (in their job or at public events), some present themselves aggressively and invincibly, but off-stage they disintegrate and need drugs and medication to get back into shape for the next competition. People who are stuck in an internal perpetrator-victim split, basically only have a choice between explosion and implosion – both of which lead to even further self destruction.

The contradictions in their feelings, thoughts and actions are not recognised as such by traumatised people constantly living in their perpetrator-victim split. I was writing this text at the turn of the year 2017/18 and wondered, how it is possible that in Germany there were heated debates about diesel emissions and driving restrictions in inner cities throughout the entire year and then, as the clock strikes midnight on the 31st December, fireworks and flares are shot into the air, producing almost a fifth of the annual total of particulate emissions, not to mention the danger to eyes, ears, and hands, and also house fires and the piles of rubbish left afterwards.

---

[5] http://kfn.de/kfn/institut/ehemalige-direktoren/prof-dr-christian-pfeiffer/

What is seen as an irrevocable truth today can be completely forgotten tomorrow. A high survival intelligence that allows a person to navigate situations in his life is accompanied by a loss of mental clarity and orientation. For someone who is stuck in a perpetrator-victim dynamic everything they do becomes more and more confused, abstract, and complicated. The person concerned does not get wiser over time but rather more ignorant, more confused, and more erratic. Therefore, it does not come as a surprise that trauma perpetrators and victims are prone to dementia in old age.

Perpetrator-victim dynamics can manifest in what is described, in the language of psychiatry, as 'psychoses' or 'schizophrenia'. Delusional thinking is not an 'illness', but rather the result of trauma-related denial of reality and abandonment of the 'I' and free will, thus forming the basis of victim and perpetrator attitudes.

Likewise, 'personality disorders' are not a 'mental illness'; the symptoms of the so-called 'narcissistic personality disorder', for example, are easy to explain as consistent expressions of perpetrator attitudes. The following criteria are listed for a 'narcissistic personality disorder' in the Diagnostic and Statistical Manual of Mental Disorders, (DSM IV):

(1) has a grandiose sense of self-importance (e.g., exaggerates achievements and talents, expects to be recognized as superior without commensurate achievements)

(2) is preoccupied with fantasies of unlimited success, power, brilliance, beauty, or ideal love

(3) believes that he or she is 'special' and unique and can only be understood by, or should associate with, other special or high-status people (or institutions)

(4) requires excessive admiration

(5) has a sense of entitlement, i.e., unreasonable expectations of especially favourable treatment or automatic compliance with his or her expectations

(6) is interpersonally exploitative, i.e., takes advantage of others to achieve his or her own ends

(7) lacks empathy: is unwilling to recognize or identify with the feelings and needs of others
(8) is often envious of others or believes that others are envious of him or her
(9) shows arrogant, haughty behaviours or attitudes

The so-called 'narcissist' wants to force relationships and love through violence, to have his personal humiliations be forgotten by his primary caregivers: "You have to love, admire, and worship me! You also have to worship those things I project my love onto (God, America, Germany ...), otherwise I am prepared to degrade you (even with sexual sadism) or even kill you." 'Narcissists' are not really concerned with themselves since they do not actually know who they are; what is important is the image that others have of them that must fulfil their desire to be seen as superior.

In so-called 'dependent personality disorders', by comparison, all listed symptoms are expressions of victim attitudes, on the basis that their own 'I' and their free will do not exist anymore:

(1) has difficulty making everyday decisions without an excessive amount of advice and reassurance from others
(2) needs others to assume responsibility for most major areas of his or her life
(3) has difficulty expressing disagreement with others because of fear of loss of support or approval.
(4) has difficulty initiating projects or doing things on his or her own (because of a lack of self-confidence in judgment or abilities rather than a lack of motivation or energy)
(5) goes to excessive lengths to obtain nurturance and support from others, to the point of volunteering to do things that are unpleasant
(6) feels uncomfortable or helpless when alone because of exaggerated fears of being unable to care for himself or herself

(7) urgently seeks another relationship as a source of care and support when a close relationship ends

(8) is unrealistically preoccupied with fears of being left to take care of himself or herself (DSM IV)

The so-called 'dependent' constantly takes a position of submission because of his previous experiences of violence, in the hope that this will result in acceptance and love. "I will do anything for you (even sexual masochism)".

Consequently, the 'narcissistic' and the 'dependent' personality traits complement each other within the one person, often in an attempt to cover up and compensate their victim attitudes with perpetrator attitudes. People with a pronounced victim attitude often seek out people with pronounced perpetrator attitudes, seeing them as their saviour.

This can be easily observed in partnerships in which men frequently assume a position of dominance and women take on a subordinate position. Or in commerce where employees with victim attitudes often expect uncompromising perpetrator attitudes from management, and equate those perpetrator attitudes as 'competency' and 'leadership qualities', all of which are further encouraged through leadership-training and coaching programmes.

This perpetrator-victim-attitude interplay is even more drastically visible in the political sphere. Voters with pronounced victim attitudes want heads of state and presidents who are 'strong', 'charismatic' personalities who are 'prepared to assert themselves'. This can lead to leadership cults in which the leaders may consider themselves more and more godlike the more they are worshipped by 'their people'. People who have not developed a stable 'I' like to bathe in the glory of others whose non-existent healthy 'I' is replaced by a magnificently staged façade, merely a trauma-survival 'I'.

What otherwise would be seen as antisocial and criminal behaviour or 'psychopathy' in the case of a 'charismatic leader' is reinterpreted by their supporters as an expression of particular cleverness or craftiness; they do not get caught when lying or stealing is considered admirable, marking them out as vastly superior to the common thief. Self-proclaimed lords, kings, tsars, and princes celebrate themselves, and refer to 'alternative facts' when reality actually looks very different.

Therefore, it happens that in many communities, there are streets, public places, airports and even entire cities that are named after notorious liars, murderers and war criminals, and nobody is really bothered by it.

As with all trauma survival strategies, the forced nationalism exerted from above causes the opposite effect: more and more people eventually revolt against it and so it leads to a splitting of the nation and the birth of separatist movements.

The perpetrator-victim split and the body

Chronic physical illnesses (gastrointestinal disorders, cancer, autoimmune diseases etc.) in my experience are the physical expression of internal perpetrator-victim splits at work in an individual. The permanent stress caused by being a victim as well as a perpetrator, and all the related feelings, lead to the person no longer being able to experience and feel their body. As a survival strategy, the body is left to its own devices, and the result is that it can barely regulate or regenerate itself because of the contradictory demands caused by the victim-perpetrator attitude. The body signals, in the form of pain, infections, digestion problems, cardiac arrhythmia and so forth, are ignored by the trauma-survival parts, or are 'dealt with' by medical treatment (Ruppert and Banzhaf, 2017).

Adolf Hitler for example had no feeling for his body, which is shown amongst other things by his distorted body posture and his awkward and erratic movements with his hands. He constantly felt unwell, had chronic flatulence, and he depended on the drug cocktails his personal physician, Theodor Morell, administered to him daily. In the end his body expressed a clearly visible shaking palsy of his hands, which, in his perpetrator attitude of alleged invincibility, Hitler tried to cover up.

Suicidal tendencies

Suicidal tendencies are a permanent part of the inner life of many people who are stuck in their perpetrator-victim split. When a mother does not want her child, the child's resulting wish not to exist is an obvious victim attitude. It is paired with deep resignation and shame, and this victim attitude can lead to suicide. Suicide can also be the result of a perpetrator attitude if the person's perpetrator projects fail and he begrudges others the triumph of having defeated him.

On the 30th April 1945, Hitler shot himself to avoid having to witness the end of his political project of a 'Thousand-Year Reich'. In this way, he kept the illusion alive right up to his death that others would not be able to defeat him. In his Will he feigned the continuation of a third German Reich by making arrangements for his successor, which was no longer relevant. A deep shame and acceptance of his guilt would have been a healthy alternative.

Nobody is born a trauma perpetrator. Studying the biographies of famous trauma perpetrators, we find significant perpetrator-victim dynamics in their family of origin and major experiences in their past where they were the victim.

Case study of Anders Bering Breivik: From childhood trauma-victim to mass murderer [6]

Not wanted, not loved, not protected – the trauma triad completely holds true for Anders Behring Breivik, who assassinated 77 young people on the 22nd July 2011 in Norway. He was born on the 13th February 1979 in Oslo. His mother considered aborting him during her pregnancy. When she visited a hospital for that purpose, she found it was too late for a legal termination. During her pregnancy in accordance with the logic of perpetrator-victim reversal, she said to a doctor, "The child kicks me,

---

[6] For the research for this case study I primarily refer to the following internet source: http://www.stern.de/politik/ausland/anders-behring-breivik-anschlag-norwegen-jahrestag-6972868.html accessed on the 21/5/2017.

almost deliberately, to torture me." Following the birth, she was of the opinion that the child was bad; she stopped nursing him after 10 months because she felt that the strong and aggressive sucking of the child would destroy her. It is not surprising that Anders' mother had this attitude; she herself had experienced unkindness and violent degradation, abuse, and sexual traumatisation in her family of origin.

Anders was not wanted by his father either, who separated from his wife when his son was one year old. Afterwards Anders' mother contemplated giving him up for adoption. Neither his mother nor his father ever showed him any love. After the parents' separation, his father saw him once a year, and his mother was dealing with her own problems, and would have liked to get rid of the child all together. She approached a social services agency in Oslo in 1981 in order to place her son into weekend care, because she said he was too demanding.

A child psychiatrist who saw Anders suspected sexual assault. When Anders was four years old, the psychiatrist wrote a letter to the youth welfare office in which he stated that the boy had difficulties in expressing himself emotionally, that he was passive in his play and that there was a complete absence of elements of joy and pleasure, and in addition he avoided contact with other children. In the course of a three-week stay in a state centre for child and adolescent psychiatry, his mother was diagnosed with 'borderline personality disorder in combination with anxiety and depression', basically in my view a clear sign that she had also experienced sexualised violence and the trauma triad in her childhood. Sometimes she screamed at her son saying that she wished that he were dead. On other days, however, it seems she cuddled up with him in bed at night. The psychiatrist suggested to the authorities that Anders should be placed in a care home; such a decision, however, was not made by the social authorities.

His father continued to show no real interest in Anders, considering him lazy, uncommunicative, and apathetic. Anders' peers did not care for him either and during his primary school years, it seems he was barely noticed; even though he was there, somehow he was not. He simply functioned at a basic level.

Neighbours reported that the 'young Breivik' was different from other children, that he was an animal abuser and that the parents of other children kept their children and pets away from him. He was left by himself and forced to look after himself.

In 1983, on the back of these alarming assessments, the father, who by now was living in France, applied for custody of Anders, but his application was rejected. In the early 1980's the youth welfare office wanted to provide a parenting counselling for the family but the mother refused. In 1990, the father moved back to Oslo, which strengthened the contact between him and Anders for a while.

As an adolescent, Anders wanted nothing more than to belong to a group. When he could not achieve that, he went a step further: he wanted to become the leader of a gang. "He tried so hard to be cool that he was totally uncool", a former classmate later recalled.

In 1994, after a stay in Denmark, Anders picked up a large number of spray cans, which he and others of his age used to spray graffiti onto houses. Because of incidents like this his relationship with his father deteriorated again, and shortly afterwards all contact ceased. At the age of 15 Anders expressed an unsatisfied longing for his father to a relative: "If one day I accomplish something great then maybe my father will want to see me again."

Anders went to the trade school in Oslo until 1998, however he left without graduating. He tried to set up companies himself and speculated in shares, but due to his lack of funds, he moved back into his teenage bedroom at his mother's house in 2006. There he spent most of his time in front of his computer playing 'World of Warcraft'. Through the Internet, he encountered right-wing extremists who produced propaganda for 'White Power' and 'Anti- Jihad' organisations. In addition to enemies in the virtual world of the Internet, Anders B. Breivik now discovered potential enemies in reality – Muslims and all of those who, in his opinion, opened the gates to Europe for them. Soon it was no longer enough for him just to read the texts of others; he contacted right-wing authors and bloggers, wanting to become part of their community. However, he was not accepted here either, another rejection for him.

That is when he sat down and wrote his 'manifesto', his very personal 'head-birth' fantasy, under the title '2083 A European Declaration of Independence'. In this manifesto, he depicted a picture of Europe without Muslims and 'traitors'. Having spent nine years writing this book, he then proceeded to buy weapons, rent a small farm, order fertilisers and build a gigantic bomb which he detonated in July 2011 in front of the government buildings in Oslo killing eight people.

Breivik believed that his act would be a signal for right-wing extremist groups throughout Europe to instigate a revolution. He had emailed his 1500-page manifesto to 6,000 right-wing-thinking people before detonating his bomb. Six hours before the attack he had also uploaded a promotional video on YouTube in which a few key elements of his manifesto were summarised, and in which, amongst other things, he was shown with a gun. He also posted images of himself on the net, which showed him as a well-dressed man in a Freemason's uniform. According to his statements, these were propaganda pictures of one of the 'most influential individuals of our time'.

Breivik knew that the next killing that he had planned would not be easy. He prepared for it with meditation, stimulants, and cognitive techniques. He had already trained himself into a certain emotional dullness through his computer games. In his manifesto, he described the young people on the island of Utøya as vermin, pests, and culprits, and then before executing the massacre he took a cocktail of ephedrine, aspirin, and caffeine.

After his rampage on Utøya, Breivik allowed the police to arrest him without resistance. During his interrogation, he noticed a small scratch on his finger and started to moan in a predictable perpetrator attitude: "You see, I am injured! That has to be bandaged! I have lost a lot of blood already!" Whilst he received medical care, he thought aloud how he could have gotten the wound. He remembered that something had hit him on the finger, when he shot a person at close range. He remarked that it must have been a piece of skull bone. Throughout the interrogation, he became increasingly lost in the perpetrator attitude that actually he himself was the victim in this event. He told the police officer that this day was the worst of his life. When his lawyer arrived on the 23rd July, Breivik uttered the insightful sentence: "If you have a great pain in your heart then you know that in order to stop this you have to inflict pain on others."[7]

During the trial he did not deny his murders, however he pleaded 'innocent' due to him being an activist, saying that it was a result of the injustice he was suffering. Initially he did not find the killing easy, but after his first murder, everything became very easy. He described the slaughter on Utøya as a book launch: "How many do I have to kill so that my manifesto is read?" During the entire trial Breivik's face was emotionless, even when his victims with their amputated limbs and glass eyes made an appearance in the courtroom. Only when the prosecutor played a film about the Islamisation of Europe, accentuated by sacred music and edited by Breivik, did he break down and said, sobbing and full of self-pity, "That is my film, my film, I didn't know if anyone would ever get to see it!" Here it can be seen how close together perpetrator and victim attitudes lie.

Breivik continued to radicalise his perpetrator attitude even further during his detention. He complained about inhuman treatment of him in the high-security prison in Oslo. He went to court in order to complain about a violation of human rights against him. Again, he saw himself as the victim.

Anders B. Breivik can be studied as an example of the devastating psychological effects of the trauma triad:

– Not being wanted leads to the abandonment of the person's own identity and the attempt to invent a substitute identity through identifications. Since Breivik was basically never wanted by any other person in his case the substitute identity does not consist of the identification with another person, but rather with something more abstract: the idea of a perfect

---

[7] "Hvis du har den smerten i hjertet, så vet du at for å stoppe smerten, så må man påføre smerte." (Seierstad 2014, p. 406)

Europe free of Muslims. With that he wanted to create a membership with a group of like-minded people for himself and prove his ability in service to the cause.

- Not to be loved in his case equally did not lead to the projection of his love onto another person. For that he would have had to have experienced something like love from another person at some point in his trauma biography, which he did not. He was also not able to direct his love towards his country, since he had never experienced compassion and loving support from there either. He just continued to be at the mercy of his perpetrator mother. Therefore, he focused his child-like love on something vague and abstract: a Western Christian World that had to be saved from the invasion of Muslims. He took refuge in the common myth of the hero who dedicated his life to the rescue of his beloved ideal from evil. This would be his life's task for which – if necessary – he would even sacrifice his own life.

- Not having been protected as a child led to an overarching feeling of threat in Breivik, which he could not see as coming from his mother or prenatal or early childhood experiences, since these were stored and suppressed in his unconscious. He could only experience danger as something external and abstract as long as access to his inner 'I' was obstructed. This constant feeling of threat, from which he was not able to escape throughout his life, forced him into activism and his cruel deeds. Since he saw it as legitimate to ward off the alleged external danger, he did not consider himself guilty and so did not have to be ashamed of his crimes.

Perpetrator attitudes can also weaken, as shown in Breivik's behaviour towards a youth into whose eyes he looked as he was about to shoot him at close range. This youth begged Breivik not to kill him. Since this probably briefly triggered his own traumatised child part Breivik 'only' shot him in the shoulder so that the youth survived the massacre.

The fact that when in custody Breivik received letters not just from extremely right-wing like-minded people, but also love letters from women, shows that advanced perpetrator attitudes cannot be shaken even by the most cruel acts. This makes clear how male sadism and female masochism can complement each other. With trauma perpetrators who escape into such perpetrator attitudes, crazy ideas and mental constructs rank significantly higher than the death and suffering of real people. Because they completely split off their own 'I', their feelings and physical sensations, they merely live in the fantasised world of their heads. They do not allow actual realities to come close to their consciousness.

6
Traumatised and traumatising societies

When many people are traumatised and internally stuck in perpetrator-victim dynamics, human collectives then also communities become traumatised societies. What characterizes a traumatised society? This is similar to the individuals in which traumatisations appear in the form of physical and mental symptoms as well as in their trauma-survival strategies. Traumatisations in societies are expressed by the overly prevalent negative social symptoms, as well as the survival strategies employed by the respective society to deal with these symptoms. Such mass social phenomena include:

- high rates of abortions; many early pregnancies in young mothers,
- many women who unintentionally become mothers and/or have too many children,
- high rates of birth complications, related to severe physical and psychological injuries for mothers and newborns (forceps, ventouse, Caesarean section etc.),
- low number of breastfeeding mothers,
- high percentage of infants that are separated from their mothers too early and for too long (nurseries, newborns given to grandparents, older siblings that have to take on the role of parents for their younger siblings etc.),
- early neglect of nearly a whole generation of small children with psychosomatic illnesses (i.e. bed-wetting, ear-, throat-, and skin diseases),
- high rate of single mothers,
- high numbers of sexual traumatisations of babies, toddlers, pre-school and school children,

- high competitive pressures at school with high 'failure' rates, effects such as depression, 'hyperactivity', or bullying among pupils,
- high pressure on parents to 'combine' family and work life in a competing economy,
- high unemployment quotas in a population that is fit to work,
- widespread poverty in all age groups,
- no proper safeguards for old age, and low pensions for a large part of the older population, especially women,
- high crime rates (thefts, burglaries, fraud, murders) and many people with even more psychological disturbances after imprisonment than before,
- violent crime and action films on all media channels; computer games glorifying violence,
- ubiquitous pornography and prostitution, with the corresponding attendant criminality,
- widespread consumption of addictive drugs and addictive behaviours in various forms (medications, alcohol, heroin, cocaine, designer drugs, excessive sports, gambling, shopping, working, and eating; relationship addiction),
- high rates of chronic physical suffering and a health system that cannot offer any effective treatments,
- high rates of people with chronic psychological problems who are not healed by the psychiatric and psychotherapeutic systems, but are merely managed ('revolving door syndrome' in psychiatric wards),
- high rates of suicide, including a rising number of young child suicides,
- a mass media that claims exclusive rights of interpretation on social and political events and so do not enlighten people but keep them uneducated and uninformed, and manipulate them,
- sciences and scientists who invent ideologies and promote them instead of providing proper knowledge and information about the realities,

- racism and other forms of discrimination – colour, gender, nationality, sexual orientation,
- high attraction of people to extremist right or left political parties and rampant hate speeches in social media,
- constant monitoring and spying on the private lives of people by government bodies,
- terror through violence exercised by large nation states as well as smaller 'terrorist' groups,
- high expenditure on the military, secret services, arms manufacture and/or arms procurement,
- permanent wars and constant readiness for war ...
- ... with the consequence of enormous and rapidly increasing numbers of refugees who cannot live any longer where they were born.

If a large percentage of people in a social structure is stuck in perpetrator-victim splits there will be numerous and devastating consequences. On the political level that is war, violence, terror, suppression and racism. On an economic level it leads to exploitation on a massive scale, poverty, discrimination, and bullying at the workplace. In the area of family and marriage, sexual assaults are tolerated and seen as inevitable. Likewise, lack of warm feelings and love in families, the neglect of children's basic needs from very early, the sexual traumatisation of children, and violence in the educational system is widely accepted as being normal (de Mausse, 1980).

Since people are shaped by victim and/or perpetrator attitudes, their thinking is extremely confused and they do not recognise the obvious logical contradictions of their arguments, so they are easily manipulated and intimidated. Since their thinking is separated from their feelings and their body experiences, they are vague, aloof, and random. Being highly stressed, they tend to get locked into conflicts because of their confused thought constructions resulting from constant inner stress.

Therefore, the public dissemination, recognition, and popularity of opinions, views, or theories are not a statement of their logical quality, coherence or truth, but, on the contrary, mere opinions that are deemed useful to the perpetrator and victim attitudes that are socially acceptable and eagerly discussed. Truths are disruptive in these circumstances and so the following principle is more likely to hold true: in traumatised societies wrong is right and right is wrong. Therefore, people are only allowed to voice their opinions in newspapers or talk shows because they confirm perpetrator or victim attitudes shared by the majority, not because they are true.

Once the perpetrator-victim spiral has gained momentum, it is difficult to stop it. This spiral relentlessly revolves within interpersonal relationships, sucking more and more people into its dynamics. This continues over generations: everyone drawn into such dynamics (simply by being born into such a system) is forced to take part and become a victim and a perpetrator themselves.

Since there cannot be a solid community between people with perpetrator and victim attitudes, religious, national, and ethnic illusions of solidarity have to be propagated, creating fragile, and constantly questioned psychological constructs for the coexistence of the group. Constructs such as 'family', 'people', or 'nation' are used to represent an idealized community of 'good people'. They serve as a reason to exert private arbitrary ideas in order to create cohesion by psychological and physical violence.

There are some fundamental imperatives in such pseudo-societies:

- Harming others is normal.
- Abandoning the 'I' is normal.
- Making sacrifices is the best way to salvation.
- The perpetrators are the saviours.
- Truths must not be spoken out, or at least not be taken seriously.

In this pseudo-society, the world is upside down: perpetrators feel like victims and victims feel like perpetrators. Because of the fears and internal chaos of those who participate in these societies, the wish is always present for a strong man or woman to be on top who is prepared to use maximum force and violence as head of the family clan, manager of a business syndicate or president of a country. Only he/she is seen as able to put an end to the arguments and bickering, make 'tough decisions for the benefit of the whole of society', and ensure 'decency', 'cleanliness' and 'law and order'. Anyone who does not participate has gambled away his right to belong to this society and will have a hard time. With this kind of propaganda, traumatised people can very quickly become embroiled in wars.

In 1928, the English pacifist Arthur Ponsonby ingeniously put the perpetrator ideologies that came into play as war propaganda in World War I into a nutshell:

1. We do not want war.
2. The opposite party alone is guilty of war.
3. The enemy is the face of the devil.
4. We defend a noble cause, not our own interest.
5. The enemy systematically commits cruelties; our mishaps are involuntary.
6. The enemy uses forbidden weapons.
7. We suffer small losses, those of the enemy are enormous.
8. Artists and intellectuals back our cause.
9. Our cause is sacred.
10. All who doubt our propaganda are traitors.

Anyone who has studied the wars that followed World Wars I and II will notice that the propaganda employed has not profoundly changed to this day. These are classic trauma-perpetrator attitudes that cause widespread misfortune and death. Anyone who expresses doubt about the official war propaganda is considered to be 'the fifth column of the enemy' or a 'conspiracy theorist' who does not live in the real world.

In such trauma collectives it does not matter that the economy is based on brutal competition, with a fantasy of endless growth, and an excessive greed for profit; and despite all this everyone is afraid that everything will collapse tomorrow ('financial crisis') and they will be left facing great misery. So to work for large corporations that can enforce their interests over others seemingly shows that both manager and employee have backed the right horse, because it is the winning horse – until the next financial collapse.

The consumption of all sort of things that nobody really needs becomes a distracting diversion strategy, offering short-term compensation for giving up on one's own will and favouring the decision-making of those with economic power. Attempts at honest, healthy relationships with other people in our work and economic life increasingly take a backseat; nobody can really be trusted in such an economic world. Everybody hides behind his mask, one hand always on his metaphorical (and sometimes actual) weapons.

In perpetrator-victim collectives, we also have to learn to endure relationships with our partners in which fear and aggression often prevail over love and compassion, and big houses and expensive cars give the false impression of a family in harmony. Instead of talking about the quality of our relationships, we prefer to talk about other things: the quality of food, our holiday trips or the technical gadgets we think we absolutely must have. If a husband wants too much sex, he can go to a prostitute; why else has this cultural phenomenon existed since antiquity? If necessary a daughter may have to pay the price of keeping a boring marriage alive and the husband at a distance from the marital bed. Many mothers give their daugthers to their husbands for sexual traumatisation. Recently a woman in a therapy group reported that her mother had bought her extra sexy lingerie for that very reason.

Under these circumstances, children are taught from an early age to thank their parents for 'giving them life'. They have to learn obedience without question, and must respect and love their parents, even though the parents are unloving and have no capacity for a healthy relationship: "Honour your father and mother". Anything else is denounced as a deadly sin, and seen as a direct route to hell not only by religious people. To call one's own parents trauma perpetrators is one of the greatest taboos in traumatised societies.

At school, children are prepared for competitive behaviour right from the start. Those who do not learn to assert themselves against others will fall by the wayside as 'losers' and 'failures'. The children have no choice but to split internally in order to manage the competitive system that is also fully acknowledged by their parents. Externally the majority of children participate dutifully, but internally they resist, turn off their minds and do not care what they were taught or have any trustful relationship with those who teach them. Others choose the path of complete refusal and end up categorised as 'unteachable'.

The whole of society fights the symptoms

Just as individuals refuse to believe their own psychotrauma, traumatised societies, too, suppress and negate the underlying causes. Psychotraumas are a taboo subject, declared to be exceptional and marginal phenomena, a private matter, that the individual is to take care of him/herself if necessary. Obvious traumatisations and results of traumas are negated, and everybody acts as though everything is perfectly normal, or nearly. A deeper knowledge of the functioning of the human psyche is limited, and seen as superficial in traumatised societies.

Identity is defined in terms of social identity; individuals are only perceived as part of the collective in which they were born, and that already determines their substance.

An outstanding example of the inability of a traumatised society to distinguish between normality and trauma is prostitution. Prostitution is seen as 'normal', even by women, since men are seen to need sex, and be entitled to it. How the women who are bought as sex objects actually feel is rarely discussed. In a society with a 'market economy' approach, in which only a few people actually enjoy their job, it seems quite normal just to do something to bring in the money. This results in the idea that prostitution, too, is a job to earn money like any other.

Since women, predominantly, are working as prostitutes, it can even be declared as an act of emancipation, and an accepted form of gainful employment. The emphasis on making profits, and governments collecting taxes from this means that it is easy for any moral objections to such inhuman and misanthropic practices as in the prostitution trade to be brushed over.

Lobbying and bribery of political decision makers does the rest in order to dismiss any compassion with trauma victims as 'sentimental' and 'an exaggeration'. When the traumatisations of prostitutes become too obvious and are exposed to the public by brave journalists or engaged charities, they are dismissed as individual fates that have nothing to do with the system. Supporters of the prostitution system attempt to distinguish more precisely between voluntary and forced prostitution. However, what kind of free will can it be, to let your body be misused day after day for the victim- and perpetrator-attitudes of others? Ekaterina, who sells sex on the internet, says: "The thing about the men paying to be with me is that if they didn't I would never agree to see them. Honestly, I wouldn't even go near to them." (Haagström, 2016, p. 206)

Since traumatised societies avoid the actual root causes of the many social problems, instead they fixate on giving false reasons. So traumatised societies are in a trauma-survival mode most of the time; everyone is permanently under pressure and stressed; something always has to be changed and 'modernised'. Members of such a society do not get a moment's rest and never feel safe; after all, something bad could always happen: the markets could collapse, you could lose your job, your money could suddenly devalue, a war could break out, and a terrorist could be hiding round every corner.

Traumatised people exist in a permanent inner state of feeling threatened, and this means that if the external stresses decrease the internal feelings of threat start to become more noticeable. When people start to experience this constant source of threat within themselves in this way, they try to divert attention by running away from themselves. They would rather focus their attention on any societal problems than on themselves.

Parallel to this over-occurrence of stress in a traumatised society, there is also a high proportion of desolation, boredom, and loneliness. Due to the emotional anaesthesia and inner emptiness that develops in many people, they try to fill their loneliness with distractions (sport, travel, media, consumption, addictions, etc ...), or through consumerism ('shopping') or through fusion with their mobile phone, the constant waiting for new messages, mail or social media 'likes'.

The different factions of a traumatised society ultimately only argue about their choice of survival strategies, for example whether:

- to loosen or tighten the right of refugee asylum,
- to allow immigration, or to be stricter on who is allowed to come into a country,
- to raise taxes or lower them,
- to employ more police or have fewer controls,
- to invest more or less money in the health system,
- to finance more or less social work,
- to privatise prisons or keep them with the public authorities,
- to loosen or tighten up on nature conservation,
- to go to war now or later.

In respect of the different institutions of society (families, school, work, press, public administration, justice, politics etc.), the choice between trauma survival strategies (for instance, the use of physical and/or psychological violence and pressure) creates even more stress and psychotraumas in the population. For example:

- through military operations in the case of soldiers,
- through nursery places for very young babies, causing them to be separated from their mothers earlier and earlier,
- through the increasing number of unnecessary Caesarean sections,
- through the tightening of laws and heavier prison sentences,

- through increasingly competitive pressure in schools, universities, and business.

Most institutions are traumatised, and prove themselves traumatising for many of their members. Being a trauma perpetrator is not questioned in traumatised societies, but is actually seen as a necessity. This begs the question, who has not been traumatised in one form or another under these circumstances? When I bring to mind the histories of the various countries in which I have lectured or held seminars, I cannot avoid speculating that the rate of traumatised people probably is 100%. Certainly not to suffer from a psychotrauma is more of an exception than the rule in any society.

Effects and repercussions of psychotraumas

On closer inspection, all the great problems of humanity seem to come down to childhood problems. The psyche that is disturbed early in childhood never really grows up, and is constantly re-enacting its traumas throughout the different stages of life. The traumatisation of children by traumatised parents continues and is persistently supported by the various societal systems. The loss of reference to one's 'I' and the dominant orientation towards the external, by means of competition in all levels of existence, are seen as normal and are not questioned. People who are traumatised, and so cut off from their proper feelings, influence and shape our societal systems. In turn, these societal institutions affect the people who function in them and use them, continually causing harm and traumatisations to everyone. In this way mothers, for instance, who were placed in nurseries very young, are more likely to allow their children to be cared for by others at an early age. Fathers who have been beaten in their childhood are more likely to consider it natural and necessary to 'educate' their children with violence. Men who have gone to war consider it crucial that their sons also do military service. In the end, it appears to be an unquestionable essential core of human groups to wage war and permanently be ready for war. Psychotraumas in a society get further and further out of hand in this way.

Anyone born into such a system has little chance of individualisation and healthy development of his or her own identity. Right from the start, he is made into a trauma victim, and even forced in one way or another, to become a trauma perpetrator. Each individual functions as a little cog in a big chaotic wheel, which has to be kept in good 'order' by an external framework with plenty of violence and propaganda. In this way, humans become no more than just elements of a conglomerate of parents, children, pupils, students, workers, soldiers, and pensioners. They are then barely able to regulate themselves emotionally because they have never really learned to do that from early on. Their objectives are defined externally for them, and so they eagerly take up regionalisms, nationalisms, and other community ideologies, as if these were their own purposes and needs.

Trauma-denying society

Acknowledging the fact that a person is psychologically traumatised is still a taboo in most societies. Nobody likes to hear that she or he is traumatised, particularly not psychologically. Many even think that it is the worst thing that could be said to them. 'Stressed, yes! But traumatised, no! I'm not nuts!'

I also encountered this issue of denial at the university where I teach. There are students who avoid attending my lectures and seminars with the justification: "With Ruppert everything is always about trauma!" Other students admit to me that it is difficult for them to attend my courses, because the topics about which I talk are too close to their own issues. Nevertheless, there are also many students who are encouraged by my talks, and as a consequence do seek appropriate trauma-therapeutic support.

Overall I see social work, for which I offer a range of courses, in a similar situation to medicine and psychiatry. The patients, clients, and customers are in many cases highly traumatised, nevertheless the professional support systems continually overlook this.

Many years ago the German Psychotherapist Wolfgang Schmidbauer coined the term 'helpless helpers' to describe the fact that the members of these caring professions often have psychological problems similar to the ones of those they want to help and should help (Schmidbauer, 1977).

In all the institutions I know psychological traumas count officially as rather rare events, mostly linked to serious experiences of violence or natural disasters. The fact that many people have already suffered psychological traumatisation at the very beginning of their life is beyond the reach of such public consciousness. I too would have never believed something like that, if my psychotherapy practice had not taught me better on a daily basis.

Often it is men in such traumatised societies who disqualify any form of engagement with their own psyche as 'unmanly', 'superfluous women's stuff', 'nonsense', 'lunacy', 'esoteric' and as a 'time and money devouring luxury'. Instead, a man is meant to be hard, 'tough', 'cool', and supposedly 'matter-of-fact'. A man goes to the gym, walks over hot coals, and, if necessary, he punches others in the face.

I have been intensely and personally confronted by feminism and the women's movements since my entry into academia. Since I wanted to be an 'enlightened man', I started to read feminist literature in my mid-thirties (amongst others Benard and Schlaffer, 1985, 1994, Badinter, 1992), as well as books aimed specifically for men (amongst others Bly, 1993, Keen, 1991, Hollstein, 1995, Biddulph, 1996, Hüther, 2009). I even offered some seminars especially for male students at university. That quickly opened my eyes about my own behaviour as a man, and I was able to look more critically at the ways I was thinking and acting with my female colleagues. Like many other men, I initially experienced the justified criticism by feminist colleagues as destructive. One could not get it right just because one was a man and not a woman. Through my therapeutic work I know now what is missing in feminism: an in-depth knowledge of psychotrauma.

Meanwhile I offer an open men's group in my practice in Munich once a month. At these days, only men can ask for a self-encounter. Women are welcomed as participants and resonators for the processes (see more about the method and the technique in chapter 9). This group is also an opportunity for me, to do my own personal work every month myself.

Psychotraumas are the reason why many men act brutally, ruthlessly and selfishly. They are also the reason why so many women act brutally, ruthlessly and selfishly – especially towards their children. Traumatised mothers create traumatised girls and boys. Traumatised children become the next generation of traumatised couples and traumatised parents. To blame 'men' or 'women' for the various forms of physical and mental cruelties generally, would only deepen the person's intrapsychic splits, and further fuel the perpetrator-victim spiral in society. This black and white way of thinking is, in itself, again a result of trauma.

How to live in traumatised societies?

Unfortunately, traumatised societies favour those who have developed the best trauma-survival strategies, those that have the greatest potential for violence within them, and those who are able to numb their capacity for empathy towards themselves and others. Lack of compassion, incessant talking and being someone who is constantly doing something become selection advantages – as long as the body of the person concerned can tolerate this. Power-mad people 'Machiavellists', 'psychopaths', and 'narcissists' in traumatised societies are often found in leading and powerful positions, and they earn a lot of money. So the question arises, in a traumatised society how is it possible for anyone to:

- find a partner who has not experienced early traumatisation, is not stuck in a trauma of love, and has not experienced sexual traumatisation, and who is also willing to work on his or her traumatisations,
- withdraw from the cultural pressure to produce children without thought,

- avoid a violent pregnancy or birth process being imposed by an technology-obsessed obstetric system,
- avoid handing children over to traumatised doctors, educators and teachers,
- when suffering from physical symptoms, to avoid being further traumatised by a medical system that is blinded by technology and obsessed only with symptoms,
- avoid being caught in the clutches of a psychiatry that is also fixated on symptoms,
- avoid being pushed into escalating perpetrator-victim dynamics by legal systems in cases of legal conflicts,
- avoid being forced to do things that are pointless or that cause damage to others in our work lives,
- avoid being sent to war as a soldier to kill others?

It requires a considerable amount of psychological clarity and determination not to get embroiled by traumatised people and their institutions into their trauma-survival strategies, and not to subject them on the other hand to our perpetrator-victim attitudes. It is not easy in traumatised societies to find a good societal niche for one's healthy private, social and work life. In a traumatised society, it is normal to see your healthy needs as actually something alien to you, and indeed to perceive yourself as alien to society as a whole.

Fortunately, however even in trauma-collectives there is still a possibility of having healthy relationships. As is shown by the diagram in figure 8, traumatised people can and do have healthy relationships with each other, at least temporarily. If both people have good access to their healthy parts (HP/HP), and consciously try to stay with them, they may be able to stop the negative perpetrator-victim spiral for a short period of time. And as long as at least one of the partners in a relationship is able to stay in their healthy part, even if the other one is in their survival or trauma parts (HP/SP; HP/TP), perpetrator-victim escalations can be avoided. However if both slip into their traumatised parts, and then start functioning from their survival parts, and nothing is in the way of a collision of the perpetrator-victim attitudes of both, the interaction will escalate fully into perpetrator-victim dynamics. The combination TP/TP often creates the illusion in both people that they are 'soulmates', which is often the unconscious reason for partnership attractions, and many marriages.

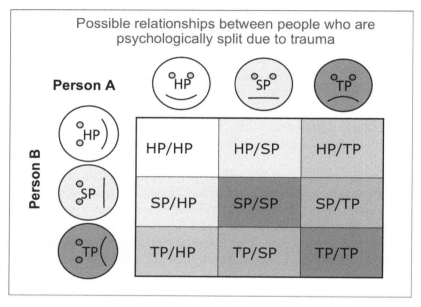

Figure 8: Possible relationships between people who are psychologically split due to trauma

With time and practice, and increased psychological clarity resulting from my work on my personal traumas, I have started to notice sooner when I start to slip into a trauma-survival strategy, or allow myself to be guided by old fears and feelings, instead of noticing what is really happening in the moment. It does take great clarity for me to avoid being provoked by the trauma-survival strategies of others, and not be sucked into a vortex of victim-perpetrator attitudes. Every situation of conflict I meanwhile experience offers me an opportunity to look more closely at myself, and see which trauma is behind my current life experience.

7
How attempts to step out fail

Living in a traumatised and traumatising society is a difficult and constant challenge for everyone. Many attempts are made to end perpetrator-victim interactions, or to overcome them. In this chapter first I am going to list all attempts I know that definitely do not result in escape from these dynamics, but instead rather escalate and exacerbate them. In chapter 8 I will discuss what, in my opinion, are realistic ways out.

Revenge

If a victim retaliates, attempting to inflict the same injury on the perpetrator that was inflicted on them, this just escalates the spiral of violence and the P-V dynamics even more. As a result, the victim himself becomes the perpetrator, and it is often the case that new victims are then created. Cultures that work on principles of blood revenge show that this behaviour eventually leads to self-extermination and extinction of the whole society. Violence just leads to more violence, stress leads to more stress, trauma leads to more traumas, and wars lead to more war. Even a criminal legal system that focuses on punishment is likely to promote further a perpetrator-oriented existence. The law and the legal system then become the perpetrator. These spirals of violence are never-ending.

Anyone who plans revenge is acting in relation to the perpetrator. Retaliation requires engagement with the perpetrator: they have to watch the perpetrator, plan and wait for the right moment, and this prolongs the entanglement. This is how the arms race was created and continues to function, and even contributes to the potential for humanity to end in a nuclear catastrophe.

Rebellion

Rebellion against trauma-perpetrators most often is a self-destructive process. The child that continues to fight her parents as an adult is never able to lead her own life. Someone who unleashes a storm of protest against the injustices of a traumatised and traumatising institution or nation will never manage to create her own psychologically healthy institution. She wastes her vital energy in a fight *against* something and is not using her energy *for* something.

The demarcation from others, as already mentioned, does not lead to a healthy identity, and so a rebel will likely cause harm to himself. He has little prospect of winning the fight against dominant powers. He often is rebelling so much against everything, that he does not even know what he would do with his victory. Indeed he has no clue as to what his own true identity actually is separate from his fight against the authorities.

The reactions of the attacked individuals and institutions to such a rebel are also likely to intensify their victim- and perpetrator attitudes. For example, a mother sinks further into her depression in light of her rebellious daughter; a father reacts to his mutinous son with remarks like, "You are a crazy unrealistic dreamer."

Institutions of power that are challenged increase their efforts to eliminate rebels and render them harmless.

Revolution

For a long time I believed a revolution against power and ownership structures would be the only way to change the obvious injustices and futilities in this world. The call for a change of societal power and ownership conditions sounded good and convincing to me in theory. However, when I looked more closely at my fellow revolutionaries and myself I noticed the degree to which we ourselves were stuck in perpetrator-victim dynamics. Our language and the tone of our voices alone turned us into psychotrauma perpetrators. Our brains were running hot, but our hearts stayed always cold.

Revolutions that actually took place in history clearly show that yesterday's victims become tomorrow's perpetrators. This holds true for the French revolution, for the Russian revolution, and all revolutions that took place after the First World War in Asian, Latin American, and some African states. Violence and traumatisation of other people remained the preferred means of control, even after the (often only temporary) victory of the revolutionaries. In fact, it actually became worse, because now more than ever they were threatened and attacked by the more powerful nations, which acted imperialistically. For the population, only the form of domination changed, not the basic situation. This makes it easy for opponents of political revolutions. In modern times this can clearly be seen – particularly with imperial America and its allies – in the discrediting of all approaches such as socialism and communism as inhuman, hypocritically putting themselves into the limelight as the upholders of freedom and human rights by means of extensive propaganda.

Ultimately, in my opinion, people differ far less in terms of 'class affiliation' and the status of rich or poor, but much more in terms of how traumatised they are, and if they are prepared to deal with that issue or not. 'Proletarians' are not automatically better people because they are poor and do not own any means of production. They can be likeable people, but they can also be tyrants who terrorise their families. Likewise, children from 'well-to-do' homes can have had anything but a good childhood: their traumatised parents may shower them with money and employ nannies to raise them, and at the same time unscrupulously expose them to their marital conflicts, and abuse them by their own trauma-survival strategies.

Therefore, the idea that the symptoms of traumatised societies would disappear if everybody was well cared for on a purely material level is not true. Material wealth has never freed anyone from the burden of his or her trauma biography. On the contrary, it seduces people to have even more opportunities to divert attention from themselves and chase a life of happiness through material possessions. The fight for material wealth, as

147

already mentioned, only leads to further perpetrator-victim spirals.

The conversion of power and ownership structures into constructive healthy relationship patterns will only happen if there is a consensus for people to use their healthy psychological structures to create these constructive relationships. This requires people to become more aware of themselves and their internal psychological life. They start by taking responsibility for their own lives and psychological well-being. Before there is an external revolution, an internal revolution has to take place. This means the dismantling of our trauma-survival strategies and the reinstatement of our true 'I' and our own free will. Only people who are psychologically healthy, who feel at home in their own body, see themselves as important and are in touch with their healthy needs, can create a society that solves conflicts of interest amicably, resulting in win-win situations. To get to the heart of the matter: we do not need a conflict-*revolution*, but a conscious-ness-*evolution*.

Forgiveness

The idea that we must forgive trauma perpetrators is part of a widespread victim attitude. By forgiveness, the trauma victim tries to take the responsibility, blame and shame away from the perpetrator. However, this takes the focus away from one's own real victimhood and one's own shame. So, once again, one's own trauma is not taken into serious consideration, and one's own trauma feelings remain unresolved. Fear, rage, shame, disgust, and pain do not get resolved by forgiveness, as they would in a proper trauma healing process, but are kept split off by focusing on the perpetrator.

It is also an illusion to think that forgiveness allows trauma perpetrators to gain distance from their perpetrator attitudes, that by forgiveness we can heal the perpetrator. Only the perpe-trator him or herself can achieve this by confronting their own perpetratorhood and their own victimhood, in other words confronting their personal traumas. Generally, however, trauma perpetrators persist in avoiding direct confrontation with their own victim- and perpetrator traumas.

There are only a very few examples of successful direct confrontation between trauma victims and trauma perpetrators. For example, there is the case of a woman who had been raped, and later managed to get her rapist to confess his action, and even publicly ask her for forgiveness (Elva and Stranger, 2017). If this can happen it is possible to redeem the trauma perpetrator from his split, because then he becomes aware of his own sufferings, anxieties and pains during his upbringing.

Reconciliation

Something similar holds true for the idea of reconciliation with a perpetrator. This is generally a fantasy of a harmonious solution, which is created to avoid coming into contact with one's own actual victimhood, and in order to maintain the illusion of a loving connection with the perpetrator. Someone who does not have a stable internal reference, and is stuck in a trauma of love, cannot imagine that he or she can have a viable existence without contact with the perpetrator. The process of overcoming trauma does not gain momentum through such contact, either. It is prevented, rather than promoted, by the external appearance of harmony. This really is only trying to render 'the old stories' forgotten. This usually does not last very long, and can easily be seen within traumatised couple relationships; a honeymoon-phase of reconciliation is soon followed by the next eruption of violence (Peichl, 2008).

The psychological splits in trauma victims are deepened even further by attempts at reconciliation. I regularly experience this when people I work with report of visiting their parents, who had been perpetrators during their childhood. After their visits, they often feel confused, have an increase in physical symptoms, and sometimes need several days until they feel better again. Contact with perpetrators causes a retraumatisation, even if the survival parts in us refuse to believe it; the symbiotically needy child parts of us still hope to be seen and loved by the parents.

Many people stubbornly insist that one day, when they are

'really stable enough', they will be able to have 'normal' contact with their parents. They keep this little back door open for as long as possible. In my experience, they only really close it if they rediscover their 'I' that was split off so early. That is, when they have worked with their trauma of identity. Only then do they realise, that they no longer depend on their parents like a child, and that they do not need their parents' love as they did as an infant.

Even at a societal level, attempts to unite a deeply split society will fail, if it is done without an understanding of trauma. Here, perpetrator and victim attitudes are merely exchanged with each other, and eventually memorials and museums are erected, but the feelings of fear, anger and shame in those concerned remain unresolved.

Saving other people

Anyone who thinks they can rescue others from being a victim or a perpetrator does not understand the functioning of the human psyche. Traumas can only be tackled and overcome by the ones who have actually suffered them. Those who are invested in helping and rescuing are more likely to be abused by the victim-perpetrator attitudes of other people, and in turn may become victims or perpetrators themselves.

Physicians, psychologists, and social workers are no more able to save and rescue traumatised people – 'their patients' or 'their clients' – than nationalistic politicians or leftist revolutionaries can save an entire 'people'. In addition, the idea of a 'people' is merely the product of the politician's own left or right wing fantasies. From my therapeutic work experiences I know that a person's need to 'save the world' stems from the child's impulse to protect his mother, for example, from a violent father.

Pathologising

To label victims and perpetrators as 'sick', and treat them as 'borderline', 'narcissistic', 'depressive', 'psychopathic', 'anorexic' or having 'attention deficit hyperactivity disorder (ADHD)' etc., does not consider the issue of their traumatisation. The concept of 'psychological disorders' or 'psychological disturbances' pretends to be an explanation in traumatised societies, but in reality such descriptions are nothing more than an accumulation of symptoms. If, on occasion, the issue of causes is raised before getting to treatment of symptoms, all kinds of anonymous culprits are accused: first and foremost are 'the genes', then maybe 'the ideals of beauty fed us by advertising', 'overstimulation through the media', 'stress', 'over-work' etc. What is collectively hidden is that it is the person's own traumatisation by their traumatised parents, which underlies the symptomatic expression of, for example, going on a hunger strike or constantly fidgeting.

Diagnoses of 'illnesses', therefore, are more likely to represent socially acceptable perpetrator protection programmes, which avoid recognising perpetration as the true underlying cause. The issue of trauma then does not come into the perspective of the victim. Theoretically, and with the current appearance of much scientific authentication, the alleged 'illness' is shifted back to the victim, as something being wrong with him or her. If there were not something wrong with the person, they would be healthy. Trauma-psychology calls this process 'blaming the victim' (Fischer and Riedesser, 1998, S. 346).

Medical diagnoses based on concepts of 'illnesses' do not prevent the person from passing on their victim- and perpetrator-attitudes to others, especially to their own children.

If trauma perpetrators are diagnosed with a pathological diagnosis, we are allowed to look at them with disgust and repugnance. Then we see them as incomprehensible 'monsters', and the perpetrator-victim dynamic that they express by their behaviour and their own victim status is not recognised. Instead of understanding that the destructive behaviour of a perpetrator is the result of their inner psychological pain, originally inflicted on them in childhood that they cannot allow to surface, their behaviour appears as an incomprehensible enigma. Now and again, they are even recognised as having had 'a difficult childhood', but it is then immediately added that 'a difficult childhood' is not an excuse for becoming a murderer.

As long as victims are labelled 'depressed' or 'psychotic', and perpetrators are labelled 'narcissists', 'paedophiles' or 'psychopaths', society will learn nothing about the traumatising causes of these victim and perpetrator attitudes. Such labelling cannot do anything to prevent the systematic strategies for the traumatisation of people on all levels. And it cannot act preventatively; instead, it subordinates itself to the political, economic, and private trauma survival-strategies of psychotrauma perpetrators in the same way that the trauma victim does.

That is why I advocate that society should focus on the psychotrauma-concept instead of the illness concept. Because then perpetrators can actually be named as such, and trauma victims would be relieved from the idea that something is wrong with them. The trauma survival mechanisms of the human organism would be recognised as a normal reaction to violence perpetrated by people against other people. The passing on of traumatisations from one generation to the next then becomes clearly visible and nameable (Jugovic, 2017). Such truths have both a curative and preventative function.

Religion

The concept of one god who, in his greatness and omnipotence is the best, and cares for his flock like a fair and loving father, is the expression of a childlike fantasy. We want to be protected by someone who also punishes the perpetrator. Religions and institutions that are based on these religious principles are more likely to legitimise existing perpetrator-victim dynamics than stop them. They rarely participate in resolving them.

A few attempts from parts of the Latin American churches in countries such as El Salvador, Nicaragua, or Brazil to concretely foster more social equality, and even promote the revolution of social ownership and power relations, were brutally stopped by the apparatus of state power with the financial and military support of imperial America. Normally religions do not have a deeper understanding of the psychology of trauma.

Spirituality

Spirituality in intellectual circles is quite a popular trauma survival strategy. Illusions of harmony and an alleged 'bigger picture' however do not help overcome specific psychological traumas. They merely ignore them, and ultimately shift blame onto the victim with the accusation that the victim has failed to reach a 'higher consciousness', and so continues to 'adhere to his or her suffering'. The ideal of self-dissolution into something greater and more complete, according to my therapeutic observations, stems from prenatal traumas. The unborn child, because of rejection, dissolves his 'I', hoping to save himself with all his devotion and love. This giving up the 'I' because of not being wanted by the mother and father, incorporates also a hidden longing to finally be connected with everything by death.

Art

Paintings, sculptures, poems, novels, films, musical pieces, and other creative forms of expression are often a cry for help from the traumatised internal parts of the artist. Trauma parts can be expressed in pictures, sculptures, gestures, and music, but art can also put a veil over the reality of the trauma of the artist. The realm of the arts and their professional interpreters can abstract, qualify, embellish, or avoid, and in so doing distract and steer the artist (and the audience) away from his or her trauma to areas of secondary importance. When these cries of the trauma victims are misunderstood as 'art', and publicly discussed and celebrated, there is a high risk that they actually negate the bitter reality they are attempting to express.

Often art is the descriptive and pictorially staged expression of victim or perpetrator attitudes. Some singers, actors, and writers become popular precisely because they portray the victim and perpetrator attitudes of millions of people in a nutshell. However, the real encounter with their genuine trauma is avoided in this way and so the lives of many artists – especially those highly celebrated in society – end in depression or resignation, drug use, delusional states or suicide.

In my seminars, I encourage students to have a closer look at the biographies of famous people and of their personal idols. When two women students looked closer at the life of Chester Bennington, the lead singer of the band Linkin Park, they immediately recognised the trauma-triad: Bennington was born in 1976, and as a child he was not wanted, loved, or protected. His mother abandoned him, his father neglected him, and he was sexually traumatised for many years. On the 20th July 2017, he committed suicide after a highly successful career as a pop star and a very chaotic private life.

The knowledge of trauma theory could open the eyes of artists in respect to their own artworks. Thus, I received a letter from a female artist, from which I will quote here: "Last summer I started to produce life-size heads and turned them into an installation with 21 heads, all 'star-gazers'. The day after your last seminar, I stood in front of this installation and started to cry. Suddenly I saw 21 pieces of me, all accrued over the course of my life, and they spoke to me and said, "Please love me!" And I was able to ask the same from them."

Since traumatised societies have little knowledge of trauma, there is a widely held view that it is alright for artists to suffer, because it leads to immortal cultural achievements. Sometimes the perpetrator-victim attitudes express themselves in such seemingly innocent ways.

Drug consumption

Drugs give us the most widespread fallacy: that it is possible to back out of perpetrator-victim splits in oneself and in the outside world. Drugs (from alcohol to medically prescribed drugs to sugar), at least for a short time, convey the illusion that everything is good, or at least not quite so bad. Drugs create an emotional illusory world of inner harmony, and give rise to the delusion that everything can be achieved, although everyone who consumes drugs knows the hangover that comes afterwards. Then due to a lack of any perceived alternative, the drug taking continues until the person's body is ruined, and all possibly stable relationships have broken down. Attempts by state, police, or doctors to take drugs away from an addict usually lead nowhere; they just fuel the perpetrator-victim dynamic in the drug-user, and in society, even further.

Rational discourse

Experts in communication have discovered that attempts to invalidate perpetrator or victim attitudes as 'prejudices', 'bar room clichés' or 'radical views' through counter arguments are fruitless, because behind the attitude is vulnerability. The attitudes are randomly chosen with regard to their respective topics according to current circumstances (Boeser-Schnebel, Hufer, Schnebel and Wenzel, 2016).

Essentially, supporters of radical positions are lonely and isolated people because of a lack of the person's own 'I'. Such people also tend to change their political camp for opportunistic reasons rapidly. Left-wingers become right-wingers and vice versa. They are swiftly outraged about this and that, presenting themselves as a know-all or jack-of-all-trades. In real situations, however, when a genuine demand is made of them, their main concern is to protect their unstable self-esteem from degradation. They cannot tolerate having their survival-strategies criticised, and they are no longer focused on the problem to be solved, whereas people with a stable self-esteem manage to maintain an overview and remain confident of getting a grip on the problem (Lantermann, 2016).

Many years of experience in my therapeutic practice confirm this too. Victim and perpetrator attitudes are fragile, even if they are presented and defended with great vehemence. Trauma-survival strategies cannot rationally be refuted, even if not very logical. Verbal attempts to refute victim or perpetrator attitudes are destined to fail. In this way, if I continue to try to persuade them further, I just remain their sparring partner. Therefore, a predominantly cognitively oriented trauma therapy is fruitless since it cannot help overcome the internalised survival dogma, that to show feelings is dangerous and a sign of weakness. My solution to not getting lost in such discourses is to ask the person opposite me, "So, what is your intention right now?"

In my experience, when people no longer need, or are controlled by, their trauma strategies, they then come to the correct and true realisations by themselves with little external assistance.

Society's failure to recognise the real problems

The many pointless 'ways out', I have mentioned in this chapter, do not lead to overcoming the victim-perpetrator dynamic in personal relationships, nor do they help in understanding and recognising victim-perpetrator dynamics collectively. This lack of understanding also cannot prevent the further development of trauma biographies within traumatized societies. The patterns and structures of the victim-perpetrator dynamic thus are not recognised by public institutions. They are not properly disrupted and managed, as the example of Anders B. Breivik clearly shows. Right from the start, public authorities and experts were involved in his case, but nobody took this child's massive victim-self seriously or reached the relevant conclusions. The trauma triad in which Anders, his mother, and his father were trapped was not seen or opposed. Thus, the development from trauma-victim to trauma-perpetrator took its relentless and predictable course with Anders Behring Breivik as it does with countless other drug addicts, criminals, murderers and suicide victims.

If a society is unable to fully understand and name such perpetrator-victim dynamics, they will play out repeatedly.

Repetition and re-traumatisation are unavoidable trauma conse-quences that every person in a society needs to understand, not just professionals. When this does not happen, interventions by the police, the legal system, the medical system, by psychologists, educators and social workers will only further fuel existing perpetrator-victim dynamics. How much mental and physical effort is exercised in traumatised societies, how many working hours are spent pointlessly and how much money is senselessly wasted in these ways?

Despite the many expenditures involved, any attempted solution to humanity's problems coming from victim and perpe-trator attitudes is ultimately doomed to failure, because it bypasses the reality of the true state of the human psyche.

Therefore:

- All wars to create a 'world empire' will, sooner or later, also lead to the demise and collapse of the respective empire.
- Within the framework of a competitive economy, all monetary successes will periodically be nullified and devalued.
- All partnerships, which are based on perpetrator-victim relations, will fail repeatedly, and ...
- As long as parents and children relate by means of their perpetrator-victim attitudes, they will neither lovingly connect with each other, nor be able to leave each other alone.

8
How can we escape?

The feeling of victimhood ...

In my experience, there is only one way to escape perpetrator-victim splits caused by traumatisation. The basis for such an escape is the real recognition and experiencing of our own victimhood. How and when did I become a trauma victim? How and when was I helpless, powerless, and panic-stricken?

- Was it in my mother's womb, because she did not want me?
- Was it because she may might have made attempts to abort me?
- Was it at my birth, due to vacuum assisted delivery, forceps delivery or Caesarean section birth?
- Was it immediately after birth, because I did not have contact with my mother?
- Was it, because after my birth I was treated without love and left on my own?
- Was it in the first months of my life, because I was put into a crèche too early, given into the care of a stranger without the opportunity of establishing a secure bond to my mother?
- Was it because during my childhood I was neglected and left by myself?
- Was it because as a girl or boy my genitals were circumcised?
- Was it because I was sexually traumatised in my childhood?
- Was it because I was bullied at school?
- Was it because I kept losing my job over and over again?
- Was it because as a soldier I had to go and fight?

158

- Was it because as a woman I was raped, perhaps even during in my marriage?
- Was it because as a patient I was treated like an object through medical interventions?
- Was it because I was injured in a severe traffic accident, and only my physical injuries were taken care of?
- Was it because someone I loved very much died in my presence?

Several factors can contribute to a trauma biography. The earlier the victim experiences trauma, the deeper the traces it leaves behind in the psyche. Prenatal and pre-linguistic traumas are difficult to remember consciously (Ruppert, 2014), nevertheless it is particularly essential to look for one's victim self in these early stages of life.

Following is an e-mail correspondence with me from a former female student: "I have completed my studies and now work as a manager in a crèche. I think about you and your lectures almost daily. You have very much influenced me and reinforced my existing opinions. I am still not in favour of crèches. On the contrary, now I get angry that there is no political action. A few weeks ago, I had a boy (2½ years old), who has been in a crèche since he was 10 months old. Since he was a baby, he has been in a crèche every day from 7.30 am to 5.00 pm. We are his family. He never wants to go home. He puts his arms around me and clings on to me. Recently he said to his mum, "Nils wants to be sad now." and hung in my arms. He does not allow his mum to touch him when she comes to fetch him. This situation was so remarkable to me. All night I thought about it. I want things to change. I want parents to become informed. I could tell you another 72,838 stories of how children suffer on a daily basis. Thank you very much for having the courage to name these things."

To look at this early time would then allow the fear and anger to be felt, as well as shame as disgust. Feelings of guilt, too, can be voiced.

As obvious as it is that Adolf Hitler was a perpetrator, as

evidenced by his insane persecutory behaviour, so far his victimhood is hardly ever recognised and named as such. Hitler's mother lost three children at the ages of 2½, 1½ and 6 months to diphtheria through the years 1885–1887. She witnessed all her three children suffocating in agony, until they died. By 1888, she was already pregnant again and gave birth to Adolf Hitler in April 1889. Out of fear that this child would also die, she tried to overprotect the boy. Nevertheless, I assume that Hitler's mother could not love him wholeheartedly and take him into her arms. Surely, she would have had the gruesome suffocating and the dead bodies of her three former children in her mind, when she looked at and touched this new child of hers. Hitler's strong necrophilia affinity and his cult of the dead could stem from this (Fest, 2001).

In order to integrate our split off psychotraumas back into the totality of our psyche, we need an approach that takes into account the developmental logic of the human psyche. In my experience sexual traumatisation cannot be overcome if the 'trauma of love', which lies beneath it, and the 'trauma of identity', which is underneath that, are not recognised. First, the healthy 'I' has to be saved from its trauma state and reconstructed, so that the traumatising life experiences, accumulated in the traumabiography, can be encountered with sufficient stability. Where there is no clear point of reference to the 'I', and to personal feelings, because of the early splits, everything is blurred in the inner world of a child.

Likewise, the development of one's own will or 'want' is required, in order to persist with the process and not give up too soon. To understand ourselves, we often have to get back to the beginning of our existence.

Some years ago, our first cat died and I wept bitterly for several days in a way that I had never consciously experienced before. My whole body shook, and I could not stop the flood of tears. Today I know that behind this deep sadness was the death of a twin that developed with me in my mother's womb and then suddenly died. I had connected to this child unconsciously with all my love and a part of me had remained in this state, even after his death. I had already given up on my own 'I' very early. There was no love for me as a child other than this relationship. My childlike loving got no response from my traumatised parents. So this very early part of me had held on to this symbiotic love of my twin who died, until I finally came to face him during a resonance process. Completely split off within me, this part had not been able to develop any further, it remained stuck in his illusions of love.

Bourquin and Cortes (2016) frequently observe this phenomenon of a deep mourning for a twin who died *in utero*. Apparently, it is not unusual for there to be a twin that does not survive the pregnancy. In my view we experience a trauma of love because of our trauma of identity, i.e. the split from our self has already taken place due to our mother's rejection of us, and if she rejects us, she does not love us.

We can only escape our victimhood experiences by being willing to explore our psyche and encounter our early traumas.

How to escape from our perpetrator attitudes

Someone who has managed to accept his own victimhood will find it a lot easier to overcome his being a perpetrator. He already has compassion for himself, and no longer condemns himself. He knows that being a perpetrator is the result of having been made a victim. I know many mothers and fathers who have understood that they deceived themselves, and did not really want their children, that they were unable to love them, abused them for their own survival strategies, and committed acts of violence against them, because as children they had not known any different treatment themselves. How could they have learned about love and warmth in their own emotionally cold family of origin, so as to be able to pass that on to their own children later? How could they have known how important a healthy 'I' and their own 'want' are for a person, when they had to say goodbye to their own 'I' and their own free 'want' very early on themselves?

Anyone who has felt their own victimhood will be more sensitive and open to feeling their own perpetratorhood and their own perpetrator attitudes. Their insensitivity increasingly diminishes and disappears. They are then able to recognise the suffering they have caused, and possibly still cause, to other people by their frozen attitudes.

Once we have our own 'I' at our disposal again, we can take responsibility for our own actions, something that was previously completely impossible. This is how we manage step by step, to feel our own guilt for the pain we have caused others. Now we can allow ourselves to feel our shame and fear of social condemnation. Then a sentence from the bible can hold true for others around us: 'He that is without sin among you, let him first cast a stone'. (Gospel according to John, chapter 8, verses 3–7)

This is how empathy for the suffering of our victims can develop. That in turn can develop into an effort to compensate for the damage that we have caused our victims. For instance, perpetrators could finance suitable therapies for the victim. All attempts at redemption that are merely in the nature of an atonement, and possibly a kind of self-punishment, are superfluous and no good to anyone.

In my practice, I see that mothers who have made contact with their victimhood emotionally are then able to recognise the traumatisation they have caused their children, who then start their own therapy. Some fathers also start to recognise that they have not had proper healthy sexual limits in their relationship with their daughters and sons, after they have felt their own childhood trauma.

Psychologically healthy children mean healthy societies

If we want to develop healthy societies, we need psychologically healthy people. For that, we first have to stop the early traumatisation of children on all levels. Traumatised children cannot regulate their feelings properly or develop a healthy 'I'. They then remain helpless and dependent, and continually orient themselves towards the outside world instead of their own 'I'. Therefore, children need to have confirmation:

- that it is alright to follow their childlike needs, to be important, and to express their feelings,
- that they do not have to deal with the concerns and conflicts of the adults,
- that they will get better and better at coping with their fears and aggressions, their love and their joy.

When children are able to pay attention to their own well-being, they become socially competent. They are able to recognise the needs of others and show consideration for them. For that, they need to have parents and teachers who are not still caught in their own childhood traumas and split from their own painful feelings. It is a fatal error to think that children will become 'socialised' through being castigated as useless and by the breaking of their will.

"What will people say!" my mother used to say when I wanted to have long hair and wear outrageous clothes during my teens. "As long as you have your feet under my table you do what I say!" was my father's usual phrase when I wanted to do something that he did not agree with. In accordance with that, I was not nice towards my younger siblings. I would force my will against theirs, if necessary by screaming at them or hitting them.

Wanted and truly loved, untraumatised children recognise within themselves the rules for a constructive relationship. All by themselves they have an innate interest to learn more about it. They do not constantly want to quarrel and fight with their siblings.

Each day untraumatised children become more mature psychologically, and do not constantly have to demonstrate their value, or degrade each other as adolescents and adults. They do not allow others to tempt them to be destructive. With appropriate support from psychologically healthy adults, they are willing and able to cooperate constructively. Psychologically healthy people know "if I traumatise another person ultimately I only harm myself. When I become perpetrator to others, it will come back to me like a boomerang."

9
IoPT and the Intention method

Access to all forms of trauma is possible, including prenatal traumas, with the Intention Method that I have developed as the core of Identity-oriented Psychotrauma Therapy (IoPT). Every psychotrauma is a black hole in the biography of a person, maintained through the personal and collective repression processes of the society in which the person lives (figure 9).

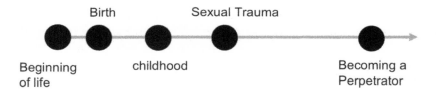

Personal and collective trauma displacement

Figure 9: Psychotraumas are black holes in a person's biography

This type of therapy, which works with intentions and the resonance technique, allows us to connect with our victimhood, and recognise our own victim attitudes. The intention is the starting point, and is devised by the person wishing to explore his or her psyche. Every intention is a reflection of a part of a person's psychotrauma-biography. It shines light onto the black holes of the trauma-biography and leads them step-by-step to a clarification (figure 10).

From my longstanding practice, I have learned that the healing of a trauma-damaged psyche can only occur from within the person. It cannot happen through medical treatment or the alleged skilful interventions of others. The human psyche is too multifaceted and far too dynamic for such simple manoeuvres. Moreover, the psyche has within itself the need and potential to self-heal, to function again as a healthy psyche that can see reality as it really is.

Because of the traumatising situations we have experienced, the need to constantly reject certain realities hinders us in our attempts to self-heal. This has to become increasingly clear for each individual person, and the resonance technique makes this possible. When other people are in resonance for me, they mirror what it looks like inside my psyche. If I can recognise myself in these mirror images that the resonators offer me, the ending of the split caused by trauma becomes possible – as long I decide I actually want to do it.

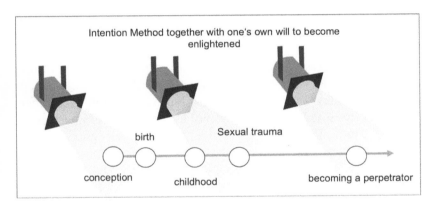

Figure 10: Brightening the black holes in the biography by the intention method and the resonance technique

Because purely verbal dialogue will not get us anywhere with victim-perpetrator attitudes, and the actual issue that has led to the splitting of the psyche is usually buried in the unconscious, I start the process at the preliminary stage of finding the intention without any detailed conversation or enquiry. I merely offer the person concerned the space in which to clarify for him- or herself which intention he/she would like to investigate.

I deliberately do not get involved in the formulation of their intention. Only an intention chosen by the actual person guarantees that they can remain open in the resonance process, when his/her survival strategies and traumatised parts show themselves, confronting him or her with their negative consequences for him/her and for others. This is the only way that anyone can really take responsibility for either continuing with their perpetrator-victim attitude that denies realities, or developing a healthy psyche, even if that is still frightening and extremely painful at that moment.

The weaker the perpetrator and victim attitudes gradually become through persistent processes of exploration, the more the denied trauma realities can come to light, and the more the healthy psychological parts of a person can assume authority over their internal world. The onset of the stabilisation of the healthy 'I', and the development of the free will, the careful attention to one's own healthy needs and the return of one's own body awareness are the central aims of this kind of therapy. In this way, the person can once again, or perhaps for the first time, take responsibility for their own life. They can gradually accept the injuries they have suffered and the fears, feelings of anger, pain, disappointed love and abysmal loneliness that have accompanied them all their life. Once properly assigned to the respective victim experiences, these feelings can disperse. It is no longer necessary to hold on to perpetrator and victim attitudes as the means of warding off trauma feelings. Those who are at one with themselves do not feel alone and abandoned anymore. They no longer have to distract themselves from their experience when with other people. Those who can feel again will recognise that as true strength, and give up the illusion of appearing strong externally through insensitivity.

Angelika: That is where I want to go

The following is the quotation of a woman with whom I have worked for some time: "How can this perpetrator, who is so deeply embedded inside me, become redundant? All I wanted as a child was to be loved by the perpetrator. Maybe one day, when

I can enjoy loving myself, maybe then the perpetrator will become redundant. Then, maybe, I will have an 'I' and a 'Want'. And that will be my life then. If I am also able to feel and notice that, or if questioning that becomes superfluous, that will be my life. I think that's where I want to go."

The practice of intention-work

In practice, the intention method begins with the person in question, who I will refer to as the 'intention holder', writing an intention on a whiteboard. Since November 2017, I have specified that the intention should have no more than seven units of information, as we now know from experience, that anything beyond that is too much for the intention holder, those going into resonance, the group, and also for me as the therapeutic guide.

Once the intention has been formulated, the single words of the intention, including any punctuation marks, are written on 'post-it' notes and stuck to name badges. The intention holder then distributes them to various group members participating in the seminar, asking them to go into resonance with each word or punctuation mark. Then the intention holder signals for the resonance process to begin. Experience shows that after about 2-3 minutes the people who have gone into resonance, come together into a certain formation, which can be said to mirror the basic structure of the respective intention.

Then the therapist accompanies the intention holder as he or she encounters the persons in resonance one after the other. They each disclose what they feel in their particular role. In this way the intention holder comes into contact with what is happening in his or her inner psyche, and finds out what connections his or her intention has to his psychotrauma-biography.

During these processes, I pay special attention as to whether the intention holder dares to show his or her feelings, and I support them in that if necessary. After all, ultimately it is only through the expression of their own feelings, especially love and pain, that the fragmented psychological structures can become integrated and unified again. Time after time, it is wonderful to see how the fragmented internal parts of the person can come more into contact with each other when the intention holder can tap deeply into his or her feelings.

However, it should be borne in mind that expressing feelings are not so beneficial in the context of the trauma of love. These feelings generally only lead to mourning not having been loved or seen, but the underlying trauma of identity cannot be taken in yet. Therefore, it takes a lot of experience, and a thorough understanding of Identity-oriented Psychotrauma Theory in order to accompany such intention processes clearly and sensitively.

Andreas: I would like to know what it is in me that I want to kill

Andreas wrote the following sentence on the whiteboard: 'I want to know what inside me I want to kill' (figure 11). The following came to light in terms of his trauma biography: His mother did not want him and his grandmother rejected him as well. They left him as an infant lying in the cold until he nearly died. The intention to kill probably came from the mother's mother side. In order to survive, Andreas had to adjust his will so as not to cry or show any emotions. He identified himself with the rejecting attitude of his grandmother and with her aggression. In later life, he turned this against himself and against others, who in his view demanded an unreasonable amount of attention.

At the end of the process, his 'I' – the first word in his intention – and his 'WANT' came into close contact with each other, and Andreas was able to witness this quite well, but only externally. His inner emergency button, which originally switched off his feelings, remained pressed. There was still too much fear inside him about what would happen if he flipped the safety switch inside him so that he could feel. As I know from other work with him, his mortal fears are prenatal and stem from an attempt to abort him while in the womb.

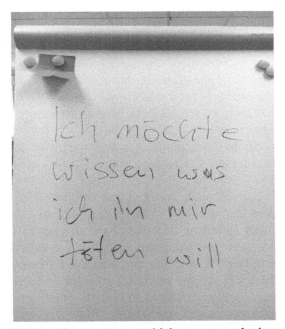

Figure 11: Intention-sentence, which expresses the internalised
perpetrator-victim dynamic

Perpetrators who trigger their own traumas

*My deepest fears are the result of being a victim myself – I was
unwanted and unloved; I was regularly humiliated and physically
beaten during my childhood by my mother, by my father and other
relatives, which led to a profound fear of violence, so that I was
also very hyper-vigilant of violent criminals outside of my original
family. I always experienced inner turmoil of helplessness and
powerlessness, and a strong urge to protect myself against obvious
trauma perpetrators such as Mr. Erdogan and Mr. Trump.
However, the more I get in touch with my personal victimhood in
my early life, and bit by bit discover the extremely fearful and traumatised child parts of me, the more soundly I can sleep, even
though in reality both of these aggressive political leaders certainly*

continue to pose a great threat to the world. Without a doubt, they are an enormous danger to the life and wellbeing of many people, and to peace in the world. Yet, at the end of the day, they are simply another symptom of the widespread perpetrator-victim splits in traumatised societies. If those two people did not exist, there would be others in their place, who would take their position in the perpetrator-victim collective that is governed by split off fears and senseless rage.

The idea of the 'evil person' is a perpetrator attitude that suggests that everything would be in order if this or that dictator did not exist.

De facto, for instance, nothing has improved in the Middle East since Saddam Hussein and Muammar al-Gaddafi were overthrown and killed as dictators in Iraq and Libya. On the contrary, the situation there has escalated even further. The disempowerment of Kim Jong-un, Vladimir Putin or Donald Trump would not make the world a better place. Even after war-prone Presidents like Richard Nixon or George. W. Bush, American imperialism still continued.

The solution is not in the elimination or the abdication of this or that trauma-perpetrator, but in the conscious exit from the perpetrator-victim dynamics of an entire collective. For that it needs, as already mentioned above, far-reaching consciousness developments across a broad section of the global population. In our current world everything is permeated with competition, and everything that exists (people, animals, plants, earth, air, water ...) is merely seen as exploitable for this competition. 'Peace' is still seen as nothing more than a pious wish.

To remain true to oneself

Gnothi seauton (Greek) – 'Know yourself!' is an often cited inscription that was on the temple of Apollo at Delphi in Greece. Aude sapere (Latin) – 'Dare to think for yourself', was the motto of the enlightenment movement in Europe in the 17th century.

I would like to add:

Dare to be completely your 'I', and dare to detach yourself from all damaging identifications and attributions. Realise that there can be no higher authority than you in your life telling you what is good and right for you. You do not have to ask anyone for permission to live your own life. It is your life and only you can live it. Only you can find out, what it means to live a good life for you.

Identity-oriented Psychotrauma Therapy (IoPT) is strictly focused on the development of one's own healthy 'I', and giving full attention to one's own needs. In this way the interest in and occupation with the needs of the perpetrators around us gradually disappears. I no longer want to be seen, recognised, understood, or loved by them. I no longer want to get justice or satisfaction from them, or take revenge on them. I realise that it is completely pointless to accuse the trauma perpetrators of committing acts of violence against me, or of not having protected me. It is of no use for me to retrospectively express my anger towards them, because if I do, I am still attached to them and stuck in my victim attitudes.

The only important thing for me is to keep the necessary distance from them, and no longer to concern myself with them and their needs. In addition, not to pity them either, especially in the case of elderly parents, who can no longer be trauma perpetrators to the same extent as they were before.

The same applies to the idea of orientating ourselves to be in competition with others. Someone who always wants to be better than and different from 'others' is not at one with him or herself. Instead he/she is oriented towards something external, having to watch constantly what other people are doing, what skills and abilities they have, always aspiring to be one step ahead. That is a sure route to stress, without the prospect of a good ending. Only the consistent reference to what I need and what I want gives me the energy to create a living environment around me in which I feel right and can be truly me.

Nobody can make a traumatised childhood different or better. We can only accept it as it was. Looking back into that time of our lives only serves us when we do it deliberately in order to collect the childhood parts that were split off, and integrate them into the entirety of our identity. For that, an 'I' is needed, which is the age I am now, and does not split when faced with the surfacing of trauma feelings. To formulate a regressive intention, for example 'I want to hold my inner child lovingly', does not work, because we cannot be both child and mother in one person for ourselves; this just maintains a split.

Life beyond the perpetrator-victim dynamic

Anyone who wants to lead a life beyond the perpetrator-victim dynamics, can obviously only do so if they can exit the relationship systems in which they are trapped. A child cannot yet leave his loveless family, and the withdrawal from a traumatising partnership most often is not possible in one day. Even when we are stuck in a work system, which is exploitative and continually creates victims, we first have to find a viable alternative. Anyone, who lives in a country ruled by a dictator, or which is at war, first has to find a way to escape the madness.

However, anyone who has recognised the perpetrator-victim dynamic in which he or she is caught, will at least be motivated to exit it, and will use every possible opportunity to do so. Their aim will be:

- to stay in permanent touch with themselves,
- to want the right thing for themselves,
- to feel their body and its needs,
- to allow their own coherent feelings,
- to love clarity of thought,
- to be able to develop constructive relationships,
- to live in healthy autonomy in a healthy community.

For me it is always a joy to witness when people manage to exit their trauma-biography and establish a healthy relationship with themselves and other people.

From the healthy 'I' to the healthy 'We'

No one else can know and feel what is good for me. Likewise, I cannot dictate to others what they should or should not do in order to have a good life. We can only learn together that power, an attitude of superiority, control over other people, a lot of money, competitive behaviour, enforced or bought sex or fixed ideas about family and partnership will not help us towards a better way of life together. In the first place, the issue is about our own internal life becoming more and more healthy, and having at our disposal a permanent, undamaged and functioning 'I' and 'want'. Individually and collectively, we have to work on our own psychological health. Collectively we have to stop continuously traumatising each other, turning ourselves into victims and perpetrators. Nobody has a right to traumatise another person, and there is no justification for it. By now I am sure that whenever someone tells me that I should serve this or that supposedly higher purpose, they basically only want me to serve their personal trauma-survival strategies. On the other hand, 'I want myself' is a programme that does not harm other people (partners, children, colleague, manager, politicians . . .). It may however interfere with their impulse to abuse me for their trauma-survival strategies. But that could also be a good opportunity for them to deal with their own traumas.

Repeatedly my life has confronted me with new challenges that I was not able to meet. Initially I tried to cope with them with my habitual survival strategies. Since often that did not work, it easily happened that I created new trauma-survival strategies. Now I am much quicker at recognising that in those situations, there is a good chance for me to get access to another layer of myself and integrate a previously split off part of myself.

To be at one with one's own 'I', to have one's own will available, to love and live in a good way, feels light. I do not need to carry the trauma-burdens of other people. I do not have to work myself into the ground, based on the trauma-survival strategies of others, just to serve their illusions, in my private or my work life. I am not fixated on relationships. I am free, creative, playful and serious, without detaching myself from reality. I do not have to justify myself and orientate myself to the specifications and requirements of other traumatised people. I do not have to subordinate myself to alleged higher values and societal principles that are supposed to be more worthy than I. I am how I am. That way I am also no longer corruptible or easily manipulated. I am allowed to make mistakes and do not have to be perfect. I choose those relationships that are good for me. I no longer give up on myself, because of a relationship or because of societal guidelines that have arisen from trauma survival strategies. Because I am in felt contact with myself, I am not lonely. I am internally fulfilled. I can make contact with other people any time, if I want to.

If the identity of a traumatised person is increasingly strengthened with the help of therapeutic assistance, the original will to live and zest for life become an inseparable part of the self. From that the desire arises for a community of people who have also worked on themselves and continue to strive to exit their perpetrator-victim attitudes and truly be at one with themselves.

In traumatised societies it is still not easy to meet many such people. Due to his observations with his clients, Georg Milzner, a psychotherapist colleague of mine, has written a book with the suggestive title: "We are everywhere, just not with ourselves" (Milzner, 2017).

We must not continue to label each other as good or bad as a way of finding our own identity; on a societal scale that is the 'trauma of identity'. I am feeling good if others are feeling good because they are at one with themselves. Every person who deals with his trauma biography and clears up his own issues is ultimately a blessing for the whole of society. Every self-confident and self-assured mother generates these attributes in her child, too. Every father that is at peace with himself can be a priceless support to his children. A healthy 'I'-reference in each individual does not in fact lead to material selfishness, spiritual drifting off, or to a diminishing societal solidarity, which demands sacrifices for the community, as some might think. On the contrary, a strong 'I' forms the motivation to develop coherent bases for real systems of solidarity.

Wherever possible, our first step should be to leave relationship systems that are caught up in perpetrator-victim dynamics, which we cannot change, but only perpetuate through our victim and perpetrator attitudes. We also have to avoid being pulled back into these systems because we are afraid that, if we do not, we will be lonely and subjected to accusations and guilt from those who themselves do not dare to exit. Here it is of enormous importance to recognise perpetrator and victim attitudes in ourselves and in others. Then we can see if a potential partner is acting out of their healthy psychological parts and really loves and appreciates us in a healthy way, or if they are acting out of their victim or perpetrator attitude, and want to impose their illusions of love onto us. Adults' childish symbiotic illusions are poison for families, friendships, partnerships, and whole societies.

Leadership by compassion

It is not only personal intentions that can be delved into and deeply explored with the intention method (i.e. "I want to have a child." "I want a happy partnership."). We can also use the intention method to examine socially constructed ideas or aims, for example "Make America great again!" or "We need an alternative for Germany" or "We need even more economic growth". How courageous it would be, if politicians and business leaders were to take a closer look at their intentions that they announce, and instead relate them to their personal biography.

When we are in contact with ourselves we recognise the victim and perpetrator attitudes in business leaders and politicians who say they will lead a company or whole community responsibly. We are then no longer so easily fooled and misled by people still caught in their perpetrator-victim dynamics and who actively fuel these through their thoughts and actions. Just a look at the biography of a candidate for leadership can quickly make it clear which traumas he or she has already suffered, and if and how much he/she has already done for their own psychological health. How should someone ...

- who has not yet taken responsibility for themselves,
- who had to give up their 'I' very early on in their life,
- who is obviously stuck in a trauma of love and, thereby, stuck in suppressed feelings and illusions of love,
- who perhaps was sexually traumatised and
- who has become a trauma perpetrator, too, without ever working therapeutically,

have the ability to be responsible for a whole society in a constructive way? That is simply impossible. They can only involve others in their own psychological chaos under the name of an authority that merely represents their trauma-survival strategies. The more power they have in their hands, the stronger this confusion will be. Here too we can apply the maxim that as adults we must not make ourselves dependent on fellow human beings.

In traumatised societies it is seen as a sign of weakness if an executive in a responsible position says that he makes use of therapeutic assistance. In my view, however, it is a sign of personal strength and integrity. I am significantly more able to trust such a person than someone who spurns any suggestion of taking care of their psychological health.

Anyone who makes use of psychotherapeutic services and takes responsibility for their psyche is trustworthy to assume management responsibilities in my eyes. The catholic Pope Francis has recently admitted that he has sought therapeutic help in his life. This fact makes him so different from and probably more human than many of his fellow believers.

What would change in a society if managerial staff would deal with their responsibilities with compassion, instead of pressure and aggression?

I recently had an interesting experience, when in resonance for the 'I' of a man from England during an exploration, working with the intention method. To start with the 'I' was split from the body, which was stuck in an early childhood trauma, and from the adult mind, which somehow floated above the body, and did not take much notice of the other inner parts. The 'want,' on the other hand, was very dominant and elevated, and wanted to be served by others on its imaginary throne. At the end of the process, when the intention holder had met the part of himself that had been split off prenatally, my experience as a resonator of his 'I' had changed considerably. I could now sense that it was up to me (as a part of him) to take over the internal leadership, but not through acting powerfully ('leadership by aggression'), but rather through empathy ('leadership by compassion').

Someone who no longer has to be afraid of her own feelings of fear, anger, rage, and shame can no longer be blackmailed or controlled by others. She has won back her autonomy. Someone who is really at one with herself, and has come to terms with herself. Someone, who loves herself unconditionally and therefore protects herself from assaults, can also live in a constructive relationship. She can love other people and take full responsibility for her own actions. She can create win-win instead of win-lose situations in political, economic, and personal arenas wherever possible, and help to make this viable in the various social institutions. She knows where societal engagement is worth it and where it is not. Blind social and political activism to soothe one's conscience or to cause others to have a guilty conscience, does not help anyone.

What connects us all

'Democracy' is and remains a form of rule, even if executed by people who have been voted in and chosen. All current democratic governments still pursue economic and national interests that are based on the principle of contest and competition. They all put ordinary people severely under pressure, punishing, rewarding, and manipulating them to participate in this competitiveness, which spawns the idea of security based on the motto: We are only safe if we are not afraid, if we are bigger, stronger, and more powerful than our opponents beyond the borders of our state, who can easily end up becoming our enemies.

However, an emotion-orientated idea of security and safety would follow the following principle: I am safe if my fellow human beings, in whatever corner of the earth they exist, are able to be aware of their fears, pains and love, and in this way are able to feel big, strong, and autonomous.

My travelling to many countries has taught me one thing: mankind's fundamental problems are the same all over the world. The mother-child relationship gives rise to the same dynamics everywhere. The potential trauma-biographies occur in a similar fashion everywhere. 'Culture' in a country is often nothing more than a different coping mechanism for the effects of psychotraumas. All over the globe numerous varieties of trauma-survival strategies exist. Why, therefore, should we continue to highlight differences between peoples instead of pointing to their commonalities?

I am the society

To conclude, I offer one more daring thesis: Who is 'society'? If we believe that 'society' has to change so that one day, we can all lead a good life, then we remain locked in a child-like dependency. It causes us to have longings, wishes, and ideas, but nowhere to address those difficult feelings. That is why I believe that every one of us is the society which she or he wishes for. A good life begins here and now, if I bring into consciousness my own traumas, exit my perpetrator-victim dynamics, and redis-cover myself. If I remain truly myself in relation to my fellow human beings around me and express my healthy needs within the public and political sphere, that is how I can remain in good company with myself. So gradually the society I wish for will develop around me and, in addition, I will become attractive for like-minded people.

References

Ahrens-Eipper, S. & **Nelius**, K. (2017). Posttraumatische Belastungsstörungen bei körperlichen Erkrankungen und medizinischen Eingriffen im Kindesalter. *Trauma & Gewalt, 4*, pp. 268–278.

Akyol, C. (2016): *Erdogan: Die Biografie*. Verlag Herder, Freiburg im Breisgau.

Badinter, E. (1992). *XY – Die Identität des Mannes*. Piper Verlag, Munich.

Baer, U. & **Frick-Baer**, G. (2010). *Wie Traumata in die nächste Generation wirken*. Affenkönig Verlag, Neukirchen-Vluyn.

Banzhaf, H. (2018). Trauma as the key to understanding physical suffering. In Franz Ruppert and Harald Banzhaf (Eds.), *My Body, My Trauma, My I*. Green Balloon Publishing, Steyning, UK.

Bauer, J. (2002). *Das Gedächtnis des Körpers*. Wie Beziehungen und Lebensstile unsere Gene steuern. Eichborn Verlag, Frankfurt/M.

Bauer, J. (2010). *Das kooperative Gen. Evolution als kreativer Prozess*. Heyne Verlag, Munich.

Bauer, J. (2013). *Arbeit. Warum sie uns glücklich oder krank macht*. Heyne Verlag, Munich.

Bauer, J. (2015). *Selbststeuerung*. Die Wiederentdeckung des freien Willens. Karl Blessing Verlag, Munich.

Benard, C. & **Schlaffer**, E. (1985). *Viel erlebt und nichts begriffen*. Die Männer und die Frauenbewegung. Rowohlt Verlag, Reinbek.

Benard, C. & **Schlaffer**, E. (1994). *Mütter machen Männer*. Wie Söhne erwachsen werden. Heyne Verlag, Munich.

Biddulph, S. (1996). *Männer auf der Suche*. Siebe Schritte zur Befreiung. Beust Verlag, Munich.

Bly, R. (1993). *Iron John, Men and Masculinity*. Da Kapo Press Inc, USA.

Boeser-Schnebel, C., **Hufer**, K.-P., **Schnebel**, K. & **Wenzel**, F. (2016). *Politik wagen*. Wochenschau Verlag, Schwalbach.

Bowlby, J. (1969). *Attachment and Loss*. Volume 1. The Tavistock Institute of Human Relations.

Bourquin, P. & **Cortes**, C. (2016). *Der allein gebliebene Zwilling*. Innenwelt Verlag, Köln.

Chamberlain, D. (1990). *The Mind of Your Newborn Baby*. North Atlantic Books, USA.

Chomsky, N. (2016). *Who Rules the World?* Penguin Books, USA.

deMause, L. (1980). *The History of Childhood; Untold Story of Child Abuse*. The Psychohistory Press, New York, USA.

Dilling, H., **Mombaur**, W. & **Schmidt** M.H. (Eds.) (1993). *Internationale Klassifikation psychischer Störungen ICD 10*. Hans Huber Verlag, Bern.

Elva, T. & **Stranger**, T. (2017). *South of Forgiveness; a Story of Rape and Responsibility*. Skyhorse Publishing, USA.

Fest, J. (2001). *Hitler*. Propyläen Taschenbuch, Munich.

Fischer, G. & **Riedesser**, P. (1998). *Lehrbuch der Psychotraumatologie*. Munich: Reinhardt Verlag-

Freud, S. (1979). *Abriss der Psychoanalyse. Das Unbehagen in der Kultur*. Taschenbuch Verlag, Frankfurt/M.

Fromm, E. (2016). *Wege aus einer kranken Gesellschaft. Eine sozialpsychologische Untersuchung*. Dtv-Verlag, Munich.

Ganser, D. (2016a). *Nato Geheimarmeen in Europa. Inszenierter Terror und verdeckte Kriegsführung*. Orell Füssli Verlag, Zurich.

Ganser, D. (2016b). *Illegale Kriege. Wie die Nato-Länder die UNO sabotieren*. Orell Füssli Verlag, Zurich.

Ganser, D. (2016c). *Europa im Erdölrausch. Die Folgen einer gefährlichen Abhängigkeit*. Orell Füssli Verlag, Zurich.

Graeber, D. (2014). Schulden. Goldmann Verlag, Munich.

Gruen, A. (2015a). *Dem Leben entfremdet*. Dtv-Verlag, Munich.

Gruen, A. (2015b). *Der Wahnsinn der Normalität*. Dtv-Verlag, Munich.

Hahn, B. (2016). Rituelle Gewalt – das Unheimliche unter uns. Ausbeutung und Bindung in destruktiven Kulten bzw. Sekten. In Karl Heinz Brisch (Ed.), *Bindungstraumatisierung*. Klett-Cotta Verlag, Stuttgart.

Hacke, A. (2017). *Über den Anstand in schwierigen Zeiten und die Frage, wie wir miteinander umgehen*. Antje Kunstmann Verlag, Munich.

Häggström, S. (2016). *Shadow's law. The true Story of a Swedish Detective Inspector Fighting Prositution*. Kalla Kulor Förlag, Stockholm.

Harari, Y. N. (2014). *Sapiens: A Brief History of Humankind*. Harvill Secker, London.

Harari, Y. N. (2017). *Homo Deus: A Brief History of Tomorrow*. Vintage Books, USA.

Herman, J. (2001). *Trauma and Recovery: From Domestic Abuse to Political Terror.* Pandora, London.

Hollstein, W. (1995). *Der Kampf der Geschlechter. Frauen und Männer im Streit um Liebe und Macht und wie sie sich verständigen könnten.* Knaur Verlag, Munich.

Hoppe, G. (2016). Abortions and Trauma. In Franz Ruppert (Ed.), *Early Trauma.* (pp. 89–110). Green Balloon Publishing, Steyning, UK.

Huber, M. (1998). *Multiple Persönlichkeiten.* Fischer Taschenbuch Verlag, Frankfurt/M.

Huber, M. (2011). *Viele sein. Ein Handbuch.* Junfermann Verlag, Paderborn.

Huber, M. (2013). *Der Feind im Inneren.* Junfermann Verlag, Paderborn.

Hüther, G. & **Bonney**, H. (2002). *Neues vom Zappelphilipp. ADHS verstehen, vorbeugen und behandeln.* Walther Verlag, Düsseldorf.

Hüther, G. (2009). *Männer. Das schwache Geschlecht und sein Gehirn.* Vandenhoeck & Ruprecht, Göttingen.

Jugovic, M. S. (2017). *Wie wird Trauma transgenerational weitergegeben.* Analyse eines Praxisfalls anhand eines 17-jährigen Klienten. Katholische Stiftungshochschule, Munich.

Keen, S. (1991). *Feuer im Bauch. Über das Mann-Sein.* Bastei-Lübbe Verlag, Munich.

Kohn, A. (1989). *Mit vereinten Kräften. Warum Kooperation der Konkurrenz überlegen ist.* Beltz Verlag, Weinheim.

Lantermann, E.-D. (2016). *Die radikalisierte Gesellschaft. Von der Logik des Fanatismus.* Blessing Verlag, Munich.

Levine, P. A. (2010). *In an Unspoken Voice: How the Body Releases Trauma and Resotres Goodness.* North Atlantic Books, USA.

Levine, P. A. (2015). *Trauma and Memory: Brain and Body in a Search for the Living Past: A Practical Guide for Understanding and Working with Traumatic Memory.* North Atlantic Books, USA.

Loftus, E. & **Ketcham**, K. (2000). *The Myth of Repressed Memory: False Memories and Allegations of Sexual Abuse.* St Martins Press, USA.

Lüders. M. (2015). *Wer den Wind sät. Was westliche Politik im Orient anrichtet.* Beck Verlag, Munich.

Maaz, H. J. (2017). *Der Lilith Komplex. Die dunkle Seite der Mütterlichkeit.* Dtv-Verlag, Munich.

Mausfeld, R. (2017). Massenmediale Ideologieproduktion. In Jens Wernicke (Ed.), *Lügen die Medien?* (pp. 134–153). Westend Verlag, Frankfurt/M.

Miersch, M. (2002). *Das bizarre Sexualleben der Tiere.* Piper Verlag, Munich.

Miller, A. (2006). *Am Anfang war Erziehung.* Suhrkamp Verlag, Frankfurt/M.

Milzner, G. (2017). *Wir sind überall, nur nicht bei uns. Leben im Zeitalter des Selbstverlusts.* Beltz Verlag, Weinheim.

Müller-Münch, I. (2012). *Die geprügelte Generation. Kochlöffel, Rohrstock und die Folgen.* Klett-Cotta Verlag, Stuttgart.

Mundlos, C. (2015). *Gewalt unter der Geburt.* Tectum Verlag, Marburg.

Peichl, J. (2007). *Innere Kinder, Täter,* Helfer & Co. Klett-Cotta Verlag, Stuttgart.

Peichl, J. (2008). *Destruktive Paarbeziehungen. Das Trauma intimer Gewalt.* Klett-Cotta Verlag, Stuttgart.

Ponsonby, A. (1928). *Falsehood in Wartime. Propaganda Lies of the First World War.* Georg Allen and Unwin, London.

Ruppert, F. (2002). *Verwirrte Seelen.* Munich: Kösel Verlag.

Ruppert, F. (2014). *Trauma, Fear and Love: How the Constellation of the Intention Supports Healthy Autonomy.* Green Balloon Publishing, Steyning, UK.

Ruppert, F. (Eds.) (2016). *Early Trauma: Pregnancy, Birth and First Years of Life.* Green Balloon Publishing, Steyning, UK.

Ruppert, F. & Banzhaf, H. (Eds.) (2018). *My Body, My Trauma, My I: Setting up Intentions; Exiting our Traumabiography.* Green Balloon Publishing, Steyning, UK.

Safran Foer, J. (2010). *Tiere essen.* Kiepenheuer & Witsch, Köln.

Said, A. (2017). *Der Familie entkommst du nicht. Mein verzweifelter Kampf gegen die Zwangsehe.* mvg Verlag, Munich.

Saß, H., **Wittchen**, H.-U. & **Zaudig**, M. (1998). *Diagnostisches und Statistisches Manual Psychischer Störungen DSM IV.* Hogrefe Verlag, Göttingen.

Sauer, M. & **Emmerich**, S. (2017). *Chronischer Schmerz nach Trauma – ein Phänomen des leiblich Unbewussten, Trauma,* 1, pp. 24–36.

Schmidbauer, W. (1977). Hilflose Helfer. Rowohlt Verlag, Reinbek.

Shaw, J. (2016). *Das trügerische Gedächtnis. Wie unser Gehirn Erinnerungen fälscht.* Heyne Verlag, Munich.

Seidler, G. H., **Freyberger**, H. J. & **Maercker**, A. (Eds.) (2011). *Handbuch der Psychotraumatologie.* Klett-Cotta Verlag, Stuttgart.

Seierstad, Å. (2014). *En av oss. En fortelling om Norge.* Kagge Forlag, Oslo.

Senf, B. (2005). *Der Tanz um den Gewinn. Von der Besinnungslosigkeit zur Besinnung der Ökonomie.* Verlag für Sozialökonomie, Kiel.

Skinner, B.F. (2005). *Walden Two.* Hackett Publishing Inc., USA.

Varoufakis, Y. (2019). *Talking to my Daughter: A Brief History of Capitalism.* Vintage, USA.

Vogt, R. (Ed.) (2012). *Täterintrojekte.* Asanger Verlag, Kröning.

Welzer, H. (2011). *Täter. Wie aus ganz normalen Menschen Massenmörder werden.* Fischer Taschenbuch Verlag, Frankfurt/M.

Wernicke, J. (Ed.) (2017). *Lügen die Medien?* Westend Verlag, Frankfurt/M.

Weiss, H. (2012). *Tatort Kinderheim. Ein Untersuchungsbericht.* Deuticke im Paul Zsolnay Verlag, Vienna.

Wilks, J. (Ed.) (2017). *An Integrative Approach to Treating Babies and Children.* Singing Dragon, London.

GREEN BALLOON PUBLISHING

Forthcoming publication
to be published 2020

Love, Pleasure and Trauma:
Towards a healthy sexual identity
Franz Ruppert

Other titles by Franz Ruppert:

Trauma, Bonding and Family Constellations (2008)
Splits in the Soul (2011)
Symbiosis and Autonomy (2012)
Trauma, Fear and Love (2014)
Early Trauma (2016) (Franz Ruppert ed.)
My Body, My Trauma, My I (2018)
(Franz Ruppert & Harald Banzhaf eds.)

Titles by Vivian Broughton:

In the Presence of Many (2010)
The Heart of Things (2013)
becoming your true self (2014)

Further information at: www.greenballoonbooks.co.uk
info@greenballoonbooks.co.uk